KETO AIR FRYER COOKBOOK

The Ultimate Recipes Guide for Cooking Amazing Dishes

(Recipes That Will Heal Your Body & Help You Lose Weight)

Socorro Molina

Published by Sharon Lohan

© **Socorro Molina**

All Rights Reserved

Keto Air Fryer Recipes: The Ultimate Recipes Guide for Cooking Amazing Dishes (Recipes That Will Heal Your Body & Help You Lose Weight)

ISBN 978-1-990334-02-3

All rights reserved. No part of this guide may be reproduced in any form without permission in writing from the publisher except in the case of brief quotations embodied in critical articles or reviews.

Legal & Disclaimer

The information contained in this book is not designed to replace or take the place of any form of medicine or professional medical advice. The information in this book has been provided for educational and entertainment purposes only.

The information contained in this book has been compiled from sources deemed reliable, and it is accurate to the best of the Author's knowledge; however, the Author cannot guarantee its accuracy and validity and cannot be held liable for any errors or omissions. Changes are periodically made to this book. You must consult your doctor or get professional medical advice before using any of the suggested remedies, techniques, or information in this book.

Table of contents

Part 1 1
Welcome to The Ketogenic Air Fryer Cookbook! 2
A Briefing on Your Air Fryer 3
Air Fryer Tips 5
Air Fryer Maintenance 6
What is a Ketogenic (Keto) Diet? 8
Benefits of a Ketogenic Diet 9
Foods to Avoid on a Keto Diet 12
The Breakdown 15
Quick Tips For Keto Diet Success 16
Low Carb Cheat List 17
Poultry Recipes 22
Chicken Jalfrezi 22
Herb Roasted Chicken 23
Pecan Crusted Chicken Tenders 25
Keto Chicken Thighs 26
Turkish Chicken Kabab 27
Tandoori Chicken 28
Cheese Stuffed Turkey Meatballs 30
Chicken Nuggets and Keto Dip 31
Lemon Pepper Chicken 32

Chicken Coconut Meatballs 33
Meat Recipes 34
Crispy Pork Chops 35
Marinated Steak 36
Buffalo Hot Chicken Wings 37
Sichuan Cumin Lamb 38
Air Fryer Nuggets 39
Beef Satay 41
The Keto Lasagna 42
Beef Kheema Meatloaf 43
Meatloaf Sliders 44
Perfect Bacon 46
The Double Cheeseburger 46
Spicy Lamb Sirloin Steak 48
Korean Grilled Pork 49
Snacks and Appetizers 50
Cauliflower Wings 50
Crispy Kale Chips 51
Quick Summer Zucchini 52
Cheesy Pickles 53
Keto Friendly Scotch Eggs 54
Bacon Wrapped Sprouts 55
Air Fried Asparagus 56

Keto Friendly Burger Bun	57
Mozzarella Sticks	58
Tomatillo Salsa	59
Shishito Peppers	60
Roasted Okra	61
Keto Fries	61
Seafood Recipes	62
Shrimp Scampi	62
Tomato Basil Scallops	63
Fish en Papillote	64
Spicy Crab Dip	66
Tomato Mayonnaise Shrimp	67
Rosemary Grilled Prawns	67
Tuna Patties	68
Chili Lime Salmon	69
Cajun Shrimp	70
Crab Cakes	71
Cajun Salmon	72
Jalapeno Poppers	73
Vegetarian Recipes	75
Herb and Cheese Frittata	75
Spicy Cauliflower Stir-fry	76
Keto Pizza	77

Keto Air Fryer Toast 78
Cauliflower Pizza Crust.. 80
Cheesy Bagels 81
Cauliflower Parmesan Cups 82
Dessert Recipes 84
Flourless Brownies 84
Almond Flour Donuts 85
Lava Cake 86
Chocolate Avocado Pudding 87
Cream Cheese Cookies 88
Part 2 90
INTRODUCTION.. 91
NUTRITIOUS SNACKS AND APPETIZERS 92
1. Hazelnut Crusted Cheddar Sticks 92
2. Sausage and Cream Cheese Stuffed Mushrooms ... 93
3. Masala and Cheese Cauliflower Tots................................. 95
4. Air Fryer Jalapeno Poppers 96
5. Keto Onion Rings... 98
6. Prosciutto Wrapped Chicken Bites 99
7. Coconut and Cilantro Crusted Shrimp Poppers 100
8. Manchego-Stuffed Chorizo Meatballs 102
9. Air Fryer Pork Chicharron 104
10. Teriyaki Bacon and Asparagus Bundles 105

MOUTH-WATERING SIDES ... 107
1. Chili-Parmesan Roasted Brussels Sprouts ... 107
2. Cajun-Spiced Turnip Sticks ... 108
3. Curried Okra Crisps ... 109
4. Red Miso Roasted Eggplants ... 111
5. Roasted Green Beans with Anchovies and Cheese 112
6. Bacon-Wrapped Leeks ... 114
7. Chili-Garlic Asparagus ... 115
8. Air Fryer Kale Chips ... 116
9. Air Fryer Zucchini Fries ... 118
10. Bacon Fat Roasted Butternut Squash ... 119

QUICK AND EASY BREAKFAST RECIPES ... 120
1. Air Fryer Ham and Leek Frittata ... 120
2. Smoked Salmon and Spinach Casserole ... 122
3. Bacon and Turkey Breakfast Chili ... 124
4. Air Fryer Zucchini and Cheese Quiche ... 125
5. Air Fryer Vegetable Hash ... 127
6. Prosciutto and Blue Cheese Egg Cups ... 129
7. Chorizo and Cream Cheese Portobello Cups ... 130
8. Air-Fried Keto Cheese Muffins ... 132
9. Jicama and Bacon Hash ... 133
10. Air Fryer Sausage and Zucchini Latkes ... 135
11. Low-Carb Air Fryer Pancakes ... 136

12. Air Fryer Breakfast Avocados 138
13. Shaved Asparagus and Parma Ham Hash 140
14. Bacon Wrapped Green Tomato Steaks................ 141
15. Air Fryer Crab Omelette 142
PORK AND BEEF MAIN MEALS 145
1. Air Fryer Crispy Pork Shank 145
2. Jerk-Marinated Pork Belly 146
3. Salt and Pepper Pork Ribs 148
4. Keto Pork Saltimboca 150
5. Pork Shoulder Roast in Madeira Jus 152
6. Bacon and Parmesan Crusted Porkchops 153
7. Air Fryer Bbq Pork Ribs... 155
8. Air Fryer Bulgogi Pork Chops 156
9. Air Fryer Rib Eye Steak with Blue Cheese Butter .. 158
10. Low-Carb Air Fryer Beef Jerky 160
11. Bacon-Wrapped Filet Mignon 162
12. Keto Swedish Meatballs 163
13. Air Fryer Tri-Tip Roast with Cilantro Chimichurri 164
14. Air Fryer Meatloaf... 167
15. Crisp Beef Ribs with Sesame Vinaigrette 168
TASTY POULTRY RECIPES... 171
1. Crisp Chicken Thigh Adobo.................................. 171
2. Air-Fryer Chicken Cordon Bleu 172

3. Air-Fryer Roasted Peri-Peri Chicken 174
4. Chili-Hoisin Chicken Wings 176
5. Hazelnut Crusted Turkey Fingers........................ 178
6. Bacon-Wrapped Turkey Breast with Dijon Butter 179
7. Air Fryer Chicken Tandoori................................... 181
8. Garlic Parmesan Chicken Nuggets 182
9. Asian-Style Air Fryer Rotiserrie Chicken 184

PART 1

WELCOME TO THE KETOGENIC AIR FRYER COOKBOOK!

Hello and welcome to The Keto Air Fryer Cookbook! Let's cut to the chase; you've got yourself a nice shiny new air fryer and you're ready to get your crispy, mouthwatering meals served up ASAP. Alas, you've taken a very productive route in your life by pursuing a completely ketogenic diet, but you just don't know what recipes match both your air fryer and ketogenic diet needs.

Well, that's where The Ketogenic Air Fryer Cookbook is about to become your best friend. In this book, I have crafted together over 60 totally ketogenic friendly recipes that you can prepare in your air fryer.

If you're already familiar with the ketogenic diet and the fundamentals of it, and/or are totally in sync with your air fryer, then you can skip the information sections and head right to my delicious recipes section.

However, if you are new to either side, I'd urge you to go ahead and look through the entirety of the book. Don't worry, the book never gets too 'science-y' and aims simply to deliver the very basics so not to overwhelm you with technical information.

You are now about to discover the start of a fantastic new diet with a wonderful piece of equipment that many of us can't be without. Please bear in mind, there is no one optimal diet, just ones that suit our lifestyles and make us feel good – and the ketogenic diet has been proven to enhance people's lives quite substantially.

So, let's get into it and take a look at your air fryer and what makes it so special!

A Briefing on Your Air Fryer

Well, the air fryer craze that's been sweeping the nation recently really has warranted the hype it's gathered. Since you already own an air fryer, you probably already know that it's basically a tool that mimics deep frying but without huge amounts of oil and relies primarily on hot air!

In a nutshell, you place your food in the basket of your air fryer, hot air then rushes around the machine and causes the food to become nice and crisp!

It's a truly awesome invention. The air fryer is great at cooking foods that are usually deep fried – so that could be breaded chicken, fish, onion rings, peas and plenty more.

From my experience, the results I get are FAR superior to that of conventional oven frying. With that in mind, let's take a quick look at all the advantages you can experience with owning an air fryer!

BENEFITS OF OWNING AN AIR FRYER

For me, I can think of a whole wealth of reasons why I decided to invest in an air fryer. Your reasons may differ to mine – but here's how I personally benefit from owning one.

Bye bye fat – air fryers operate almost completely through cooking your food with hot air, and not oil. This results in a huge decrease in the fat in your food that you'd usually endure with conventional frying.

Weight loss – reducing the oil you intake also equates to a reduction in the calories you consume. This is GREAT if you're looking to lose weight but don't want to give up your favorite foods that are usually laden in fat.

Less mess – the air fryer is a very compact little machine, ideal for those of us with small areas to work with. Not only does this help in terms of surface area covered, but also, cooking your foods with no fat results in a lot less greasy areas in the kitchen.

Easy to clean – the air fryer has been specifically designed with nonstick components, which makes cleaning the device an absolute breeze. You can dishwash all parts of the air fryer too!

A real time saver – without a doubt one of the most positive factors to owning an air fryer is the time it saves. There are not many devices in existence that fry, grill, bake and roast while given you healthy food as a result.

AIR FRYER TIPS

I've not been using the air fryer for THAT long, but long enough to feel as if I can share some great tips for those of you just getting started. There is obviously a whole wealth of information online that you can look up, however, these are my personal favorite and most useful tips to date!

Tip 1 – don't let it get too busy in there. For the air fryer to work at an optimal rate, there needs to be enough 'room' inside the basket, so the air can circulate better and cook food better.

Tip 2 – just a little shake. While it's not a necessity, it is a good idea to shake the basket halfway through cooking, just to make sure the food gets slightly repositioned and cooks evenly.

Tip 3 – a regular wash. Even though the air fryer is incredibly easy to look after, it's more than likely going to be a real staple in your food preparations – and therefore needs regular washing. Every couple of weeks should be enough to keep things functioning perfectly.

Tip 4 – you can skip the preheat. Granted, the preheat only takes 4-5 minutes, however, you don't need to do this – you can simply add a couple minutes onto the recipes cooking time and get the same result.

Tip 5 – eating for one? To save time on cleaning your fryer after small cook-jobs, you can lay a piece of aluminum foil on the bottom of the frying tray and place your food on that. If you're just making a small amount in your fryer, this is ideal for saving time on loading up your dishwasher all the time.

AIR FRYER MAINTENANCE

As previously stated, the air fryer is very easy to look after. However, it is indeed a piece of electrical equipment and therefore needs proper maintenance to run in an optimal way and avoid any damage. So, in this section of the book, let's look at how you can look after your air fryer to keep it running smoothly.

Feel free at any point to move onto the recipes!

Wash it - an obvious fundamental to maintaining your machine is to make sure you are washing it every couple of weeks at least.

Check your cords - Never plug in a cord that is looking frail. Always check the condition of the cord before starting up your air fryer to make sure it's in good condition.

Give her some space – Make sure you don't have your air fryer too close to any other pieces of equipment. For the fryer to vent heat correctly, you should allow 4-inches of area space around all sides of the machine.

Check all over – After every 4 or 5 sessions with your air fryer, just give each component a quick check over to make sure everything is OK. If you notice any issues, you should contact the manufacturer regarding a placement part.

Use your nose – Some foods can leave a nasty lingering smell if they aren't dealt with and can affect the aroma of foods that are cooked in the future. Have a smell of your fryer after each use to determine whether you need to wash it or not.

Pan won't fit – If you ever notice that the pan doesn't slide smoothly into the air fryer, it's probably because you have too much food stuffed in there. Lighten the load and try again.

Read the manual – As boring as it is, nobody knows better than the product manufacturer, so read the manual that comes with your air fryer before setting it up.

Store it properly – Never store the fryer while it's still hot or plugged in. Make sure it's cooled down completely before storing it in an upright, stable position.

WHAT IS A KETOGENIC (KETO) DIET?

The ketogenic diet, typically shortened to 'keto', is based around eating foods that are low in carbs and increasing your fat intake. The theory here is that your body will use the fats as energy instead of carbs.

Why do that though?

In a nutshell, after a few days of sticking to a ketogenic diet, your body goes into a state called ketosis – which is what happens when you void yourself of carbohydrates.

And then when?

Your body then starts producing ketones which you then use in place of missing carbs, allowing you to burn more fat. This whole process is geared toward helping the body lose weight faster.

To help summarize the above without getting too technical: the keto diet, after practicing it for a few days, allows your body to tap into your fat stores and uses them as fuel.

The ketogenic diet was originally introduced into people's diets way back in the 1920s but was used primarily to help treat people for diabetes and epilepsy. However, modern trends use this technique primarily as a method to burn fat much quicker than conventional dieting.

The trend has taken off massively in recent years, mainly due to celebrities preaching the diet along with fitness experts.

Benefits of a Ketogenic Diet

Controversy has always surrounded low carb diets and the effects on the body. However, there have been plenty of human studies conducted using low carb diets that have produced very promising outcomes.

Here are just a few of the reported benefits.

Weight loss – quite possibly the number one reason people start following the keto diet, is weight loss. Not only does voiding your body of carbs help you burn off fat, but you'll also be eating foods that are much lower in calories, which is equally as important for weight loss.

Appetite suppression – pretty important when dieting. Hunger can be an absolute nightmare, and often leads to binging on junk food. When we cut carbs from our body, we tend to replace them with foods high in protein and fat, which in turn leads to feeling much more satisfied while consuming less.

Reduced blood sugar and insulin levels – After eating carbohydrates, they break down inside our body into 'simple sugars' inside our digestive tract. This causes a rise in blood sugar levels when they enter the bloodstream. High blood sugars are toxic and cause your body to produce a hormone called insulin. Insulin 'tells' your body it's time to bring the simple sugars into our cells to either store them or burn them off.

A lot of people have a problem with this process, where it's harder for the body to bring blood sugar into cells. This ultimately can lead to type 2 diabetes.

By cutting out carbs, or following a ketogenic diet, you remove any need for insulin, which in turn solves this issue that at least 300 million people suffer from.

Blood pressure can go down – high blood pressure can bring about many diseases later in life, including heart disease. A low-carb or keto diet has been proven to help lower your blood pressure as thus lessen the risk of diseases.

More energy – During ketosis, your body uses fat as an energy source that will ultimately never run out, which means you'll find that you have a lot more energy during the day, and even enjoy a lifestyle that doesn't involve craving midday naps.

FOODS TO AVOID ON A KETO DIET

The following lists are going to be an absolute Godsend when it comes to starting your new diet. Let's look at the main culprits when it comes to slowing down your keto progressions.

Sugar – quite possibly the biggest no-no on the list. Unfortunately, sugar is found in a hell of a lot of foods these days. This is usually what people struggle to reduce the most in their diets.

Sugar is found in candy, cookies, chocolate, donuts, ice cream, cereals, milk, vitamin water, cakes and pretty much any other 'unhealthy' food that comes to mind.

Please bear in mind that the keto diet doesn't mean that you must have ZERO sugar per day. It's in almost everything we eat and won't be avoided. You need to think more so about the ADDITIONAL sugar that's getting added to your diet. Some of my recipes have TINY amounts of sugar in them that you can easily fit into your macros. Just be careful with it.

Starches – all the 'carby' foods you can think of are at risk of slowing your keto diet down. These include rice, bread and pasta as the obvious trio.

Beer – sorry to say that beer is full of carbs and will have to be limited on your new diet. There are some lower-carb beers that do exist if you crave it.

Fruit – not as bad as it is typically seen as a health food – however, fruits are indeed packed with sugar and should be limited on a keto diet.

Please note again: you shouldn't mistake the keto diet as a NO CARB diet, when, it's a LOW CARB one. As a rough guide to how many carbs you can allow in your diet, you'll want to look between 20 and 50 grams per day. Obviously the closer to 20 grams you get, the more success you'll have.

With that briefing in mind, here's a list I've created that outlines over 100 foods you may want to avoid when going keto.

100+ Foods To Avoid

Grains: Wheat, oats, barley, rice, rye, corn, quinoa, millet, sorghum, bulgur, amaranth, sprouted grains, buckwheat. Any breads and pastas made from these foods also.

Beans and legumes: Kidney beans, chickpeas, black beans, lentils, green peas, lima beans, pinto beans, white beans, cannellini beans, fava beans, black-eyed beans

Fruits: Bananas, pineapples, apples, papaya, grapes, oranges, mangos, tangerines, fruit juices, smoothies, dried fruits, fruit syrups, fruit concentrates

Vegetables: Yams, sweet potatoes, carrots, parsnips, peas, yucca, corn, cherry tomatoes

Sugars: Honey, agave nectar, maple syrup, raw sugar, cane sugar, high-fructose corn syrup, turbinado sugar

Protein: Milk, butter substitutes, cream cheese, evaporated milk, whipped topping, low-fat yogurts

Fats: Soybean oil, peanut oil, sesame oil, sunflower oil, safflower oil, grapeseed oil, corn oil, canola oil

Drinks: Beer, wines, cocktails, mixers, flavored liquors, sodas, diet sodas, fruit juice, smoothies, coffee/tea with added sweetener, sweetened milk products

The Breakdown

With the above lists in mind, let's look at what kind of percentages you want to aim for with your macronutrients to stay in a ketosis state.

Carbs: As we already know, the keto diet is heavily based on reducing carbs, therefore we want to look at carbs making up around **5-10%** of our daily intake of food.

Fat: Now our primary source of energy, we want to start upping the fat intake in our diet. We need our fat intake to take up around **70-80%** of our daily intake.

Protein: Unless you're looking to win the next Mr. Olympia, you don't need to worry about consuming too much protein. A moderate amount of around **20-25%** each day should suffice.

This doesn't mean that you must stick EXACTLY to the numbers and foods recommended in this book, however, just be aware that swaying off course too often will take you out of a ketosis state and reverse the progress – try your best to cut the foods out of your diet I've listed and stick to the percentages above.

Quick Tips For Keto Diet Success

Quick tips are great for lazy people like me who don't want to learn all the 'sciencey' malarkey that goes behind certain diets. Let's look at my top tips for success with the keto diet.

Stop eating out – eating out regularly at restaurants or takeaways is the easiest way to ruin your keto diet. Restaurant and takeaway foods are PACKED full of calories and carbs. The problem with this type of food is that it's not immediately obvious what you are consuming. The bulk of your food should come from homemade recipes!

If it's in the house, you'll eat it – quite possibly my favorite tip in this list. It may seem obvious, but it works very well. Don't stock your cabinets full of foods you know you shouldn't have. If they exist in the house, chances are at some point you will consume it, so don't buy the food in the first place. Stay strong.

Look at what you're eating – again, look at what you're eating. Check the packs of the food for carbs and make sure they fit into your daily allowance of carbohydrates.

Social support – the keto diet has now become so popular that you are never going to be alone with your quest for superior health. There are now hundreds of forums and groups online you can join and participate in. These are extremely handy for when you have questions or just want some support when getting started.

Be prepared for changes – when switching diets, your body goes through a lot of changes and you need to be mentally prepared for this to potentially happen when going low-carb. During your first few days of keto, you may experience some flu-like symptoms. Just make sure you drink plenty of water and healthy foods – it will pass. Always get seen to by a doctor if you're unsure.

Meal prep if you can – preparing your meals for the entire week is a great way to ensure you stick to your new diet. Trying to take your diet as and when it comes almost nearly always ends up in binge eating. Fail to plan, plan to fail!

Low Carb Cheat List

We've already looked at what we can't eat, so let's now look at what we can eat. I've created this cheat list of low carb foods, so you can refer to it at any given point for help when creating meals or snacking.

Replace flavored yogurt with: coconut milk yogurt, sour cream, full fat cottage cheese, full fat Greek yogurt

Replace cereals with: Salted caramel pork rind cereal, toasted nuts, flax granola, chia pudding

Replace oatmeal with: Cinnamon roll oatmeal, cauliflower, chia seed, flax meal oatmeal

Replace pancakes and waffles with: Peanut butter pancakes, cream cheese pancakes, almond flour waffles

Replaces egg whites: Whole eggs

Replace burger and fries: Steak and vegetables, burger with no bun

Replace typical pizza: Mozzarella cheese dough pizza, pizza casserole

Replace bread crust fried chicken with: Pork Rind and Parmesan crust

Replace processed soups with: Pumpkin soup, enchilada chicken soup

Replace Chinese takeaway with: Low-carb sweet and sour chicken

Replace rice with: Cauliflower rice

Replace mashed potatoes with: Cauliflower mashed potatoes

Replace burritos and tacos with: Flax tortillas, taco salad, psyllium husk tortillas

Replace bread and sandwiches with: Lettuce wraps, flax seed wraps, psyllium husk wraps

Replaces cookies with: Peanut butter cookies, low-carb cookies

Replace crackers with: Chia seed crackers, flaxseed crackers

Replace candy with: Mug cakes, fat bombs

Replace soda and fruit juice with: Smoothies, water, tea

Replace coffee with: Nothing, keep drinking it but just use Stevia as a sweetener!

Replace cocktails with: Dry wine, liquor

Replace ice cream with: Avocado ice cream, low-carb sorbet

Replace brownies with: Low-carb macadamia nut brownies, avocado brownies, almond flour brownies

Replace any pie crust with: Nut-based crusts

Replace custard with: Pots de Crème

Replace flour with: Almond flour

Replace breadcrumbs with: Pork rinds

Replace margarine and veg oil with: Butter, coconut oil

Replace sugar with: Stevia, erythritol

Replace chocolate with: Baker's chocolate, dark chocolate

Replace fruits with: Extracts

Replace cornstarch with: Xanthan gum

Replace high carb veg with: Dried spices

And there you have it, the complete cheat sheet for a ketogenic diet. It's a good idea to refer to this when you're not quite sure what to replace certain foods with – chances are it's on this list.

How to Reach Ketosis Faster

Your goal with the ketogenic diet is to reach a state of ketosis. Here are a few tips on how to reach that state faster. Typically for your body to adjust and start up in a state of ketosis, it can take between 2 days and a week. However, the sooner, the better!

Carbs go down – The most important and most obvious way to reach ketosis faster is by making sure your carbs are going DOWN. You won't ever reach the state of ketosis while your carbs are high, so you must make sure you are heading toward 20grams a day. ALL the recipes in this book are lower than 10g.

Exercise – Becoming more active in your daily life can help you enter ketosis quicker. Alongside a lower carb intake, exercise helps your body increase its production of ketones which leads to entering a state of ketosis faster.

Up the fat – A lot of people fear fat, with the assumption that eating fat, makes you fat – it doesn't! Consuming more calories than you burn off, makes you fat. Getting healthy fats into your system will help you enter a state of ketosis quicker.

Mini fast – A lot of people have reported success on doing miniature fasts, where you simply cut your calories to around 1000 a day and use fats to make up most of that calorie count. This combo has helped a lot of people reach ketosis faster.

Stay hydrated and get your sleep – A lot of people will find that when cutting carbs that they soon become dehydrated. Dehydration can cause a whole host of issues and even affect your sleep which is vital for overall health – so make sure you get your water in.

Poultry Recipes

Chicken Jalfrezi

Ingredients (serves 4)

1 lb boneless skinless chicken thighs, cut into medium size pieces
1 cup onions, chopped
2 cups bell peppers, chopped
2 tablespoons oil
1 tsp salt
1 tsp turmeric
1 tsp garam masala
1 tsp cayenne

Sauce:

¼ cup tomato sauce
1 tablespoon water
1 tsp garam masala
½ tsp salt
½ tsp cayenne

Instructions

1. Mix the chicken, pepper, onions, oil, salt, garam masala, cayenne and turmeric into a large sized bowl

2. Now add your chicken and veg to your air fryer basket

3. Cook in your air fryer for 15 mins on a heat setting of 360f. It's a good idea to toss or stir half way through the cook!

4. During the cooking period, you can make your sauce. Combine the tomato sauce, garam masala, salt, water and cayenne into a microwavable bowl.

5. Set this in your microwave and give it a 60 second blast, stir halfway and after. Set aside for now.

6. Take your chicken from the air fryer along with the veg and place in a large bowl.

7. Pour the prepared sauce evenly over the chicken and veg. Now toss the chicken and veg to it's all covered in sauce.

8. Serve with cauliflower rice or a side salad!

Carbs: 9g Fiber:3g Fat: 12g Sugar 4g: Protein: 20g

HERB ROASTED CHICKEN

Ingredients **(serves 4)**

2 tablespoons ghee
½ tsp paprika
½ tsp salt

½ tsp dried thyme
¼ tsp dried rosemary
¼ tsp garlic powder
¼ tsp black pepper
Lemon wedges
2 bone-in skin-on chicken breast halves

Instructions

1. Combine the salt, butter, thyme, paprika, garlic powder, rosemary and black pepper in a small bowl and stir thoroughly. This is your herb butter.

2. Loosen skin on each chicken breast, separate it from the flesh leaving it attached at the thick end of each breast. Rub a quarter of your herb butter onto each breast. Now lightly press skin back onto each of the chicken breasts before rubbing the rest of your herb butter onto the skin of the breast.

3. Add the chicken to your air fryer, setting it to 375f. Cook for 25 minutes.

4. Leave the chicken to one side for 10 minutes before serving with lemon wedges

Carbs: 2g Fat: 20g Saturated Fat: 10g Protein: 28g

PECAN CRUSTED CHICKEN TENDERS

Ingredients **(serves 4)**

1 lb chicken tenders
1 tsp salt
1 tsp pepper
¼ cup ground mustard
½ tsp smoked paprika
2 tablespoons sugar-free maple syrup
1 cup crushed pecans

Instructions

1. Place the chicken tenders into a medium sized bowl and add the pepper, salt and paprika. Mix until chicken is well coated

2. Now add mustard and honey. Mix thoroughly.

3. Coat the chicken in the crushed pecans by rolling the chicken around in them. You can place the pecans on a flat surface if this helps, just make sure the entirety of the chicken tenders are covered.

4. Add the now covered chicken tenders to your air fryer basket and cook for 12 minutes at 350f until the chicken is cooked and the pecans give off a brown/gold appearance.

5. Serve and enjoy!

Carbs: 7g Fiber:3g Fat: 21g Saturated Fat: 3g Sugar 3g: Protein: 20g

KETO CHICKEN THIGHS

Ingredients (serves 4)

4 boneless chicken thighs
3 tablespoons Parmesan cheese, grated
1/3 cup almond flour
1 tsp paprika
1 tsp dried mixed herbs
½ tsp Cajun seasoning

Instructions

1. In a medium sized bowl, mix together the cheese, herbs, paprika, almond flour and Cajun.

2. Use a cooking spray to cover both sides of all 4 chicken thighs (don't go mad here, just cover it lightly)

3. Now cover the chicken in the above mixture, making sure it's coated evenly and all over.

4. Add the chicken to your air fryer, making sure there is room between each thigh.

5. Cook for 16-18 minutes at 390f before serving. Please always make sure the chicken is cooked properly before serving.

Carbs: 5g Fiber: 4g Fat: 40g Saturated Fat: 4g Protein: 25g

TURKISH CHICKEN KABAB

***Ingredients* (serves 6)**

1 lb boneless skinless chicken thighs, cut into 4 pieces
¼ cup Greek yogurt
1 tablespoon tomato paste
1 tablespoon minced garlic
1 tablespoon veg oil
1 tablespoon lemon juice
1 tsp ground cumin
1 tsp salt
1 tsp paprika
½ tsp black pepper
½ tsp cayenne pepper
½ tsp ground cinnamon

Instructions

1. Mix together the yogurt, tomato paste, garlic, veg oil, lemon juice, salt, paprika, cumin, black pepper, cinnamon and cayenne pepper into a large bowl until combined nicely.

2. Add in chicken pieces and mix until there are covered completely in the marinade.

3. Marinade for 30 minutes

4. Remove from marinade and add the chicken to your air fryer, giving each piece plenty of space.

5. Cook chicken for 10 mins at 370f

6. Flip chicken over and fry for another 5 mins at 370f

7. Serve

Carbs: 5g Fiber: 3g Fat: 20g Saturated Fat: 6g Protein: 20g

TANDOORI CHICKEN

Ingredients (serves 4)

1 lb chicken tenders
¼ cup Greek yogurt
1 tablespoon minced garlic
1 tablespoon minced ginger
1 tsp salt
¼ cup cilantro
1 tsp cayenne pepper
1 tsp garam masala
1 tsp turmeric
1 tsp sweet smoked paprika
1 tablespoon ghee, for basting
2 tsps lemon juice, for finishing
2 tablespoons chopped cilantro, for garnishing

Instructions

1. Mix all ingredients, EXCEPT for lemon juice, 2 tablespoons cilantro and basting oil into a large bowl.

2. Lay the covered chicken pieces into your air fryer rack in a single layer.

3. Use a brush to baste the chicken with the ghee on one side

4. Cook chicken for 12-14 minutes at a temperate of 350F

5. When time is up, flip chicken over, baste other side and cook for another 5 minutes

6. Check with meat thermometer for a temp of 165F. Now remove the chicken onto a plate and add lemon juice and chopped cilantro.

7. Serve!

Carbs: 3g Fiber: 3g Fat: 10g Saturated Fat: 3g Protein: 20g

CHEESE STUFFED TURKEY MEATBALLS

Ingredients **(serves 2)**

1 lb lean ground turkey
4 oz pepper jack cheese
1 egg
2 cloves garlic, minced
½ tsp salt
½ tsp pepper

Instructions

1. Cut cheese into cubes. Don't make these too big – around 1 inch by 1 inch should be fine.

2. In a medium sized bowl, mix together the turkey, garlic, egg, salt and pepper until well formed.

3. With this mixture, wrap small amounts around the cheese. Only use one piece of cheese per ball you make. Make as many as you can from the food you have!

4. Add to air fryer basket and cook for 12 minutes at a temperate of 370F.

5. Serve!

Carbs: 3g Fiber: 2g Fat: 12g Saturated Fat: 4g Protein: 20g

Chicken Nuggets and Keto Dip

***Ingredients* (serves 4)**

1 skinless chicken breast
Pinch of salt
1 tsp sesame oil
½ tsp ground ginger
¼ cup coconut flour
4 egg whites
6 tablespoons toasted sesame seeds
Cooking spray (whichever you prefer)

Dip ingredients:

2 tablespoon creamy almond butter
1 tablespoon water
2 tsp rice vinegar
4 tsp coconut aminos
1 tsp Sriracha
½ tsp ground ginger
½ tsp monkfruit

Instructions

1. Preheat air fryer for 10 mins at 400F.

2. Cut chicken into nugget-shaped pieces, dry them, then toss in a bowl with sesame oil and salt.

3. Add the ground ginger and coconut flour into a large Ziploc bag and shake. Now add the chicken pieces and shake until fully covered.

4. Now add eggs whites to a bowl and place the chicken in them, tossing until covered.

5. Take another Ziploc bag and add in the sesame seeds. Get rid of any excess egg from the chicken then add each piece, shaking until covered.

6. Spray your air fryer with oil, then add the chicken nuggets, making sure they aren't crowded. If you need to do this in more than one batch, then do so.

7. Cook in the air fryer for 6 mins, flip nuggets, then cook for another 5 minutes until they look crispy on the outside.

8. As the nuggets are cooking, simply whisk together all the dip ingredients until smooth, then serve together!

Carbs: 9.5g Fiber: 5g Fat: 12g Saturated Fat: 1.2g Protein: 25g

Lemon Pepper Chicken

Ingredients (serves 4)

1 chicken breast
2 lemons rind and juice
1 tsp garlic puree
1 tablespoon chicken seasoning
Black peppercorns
Salt and pepper

Instructions

1. Preheat air fryer to 355F.

2. Place a sheet of silver foil onto your worktop. Add all the seasonings except the chicken seasonings, and lemon rind to this.

3. On a chopping board, remove any fat from the chicken and season each side with some salt and pepper. Now rub the chicken seasoning onto both sides.

4. Place chicken into the silver foil and allow the seasoning to fully cover the chicken.

5. Seal the foil around the chicken TIGHT then place into your air fryer, cooking for 15 mins.

6. Make sure you check the middle of the chicken before servings.

7. Serve!

Carbs: 9.5g Fiber: 6g Fat: 3g Saturated Fat: 1g Protein: 13g

CHICKEN COCONUT MEATBALLS

Ingredients (serves 4)

1 lb ground chicken

2 green onions
½ cup cilantro
1 tablespoon hoisin sauce
1 tablespoon soy sauce
1 tsp Sriracha
1 tsp sesame oil
¼ cup shredded coconut (unsweetened if possible)
Salt and pepper

Instructions

1. In a large bowl mix all the ingredients together until a wet and sticky mixture is formed

2. Make 6-8 balls out of the mixture and drop them into your air fryer basket

3. Cook in fryer at 350f for around 10 mins, flipping them halfway through to make sure they are getting fully cooked

4. Brown these off in batches at 400f for a couple minutes or until they are indeed browned.

Carbs: 3g Fiber: 3g Fat: 15g Saturated Fat: 6g Protein: 21g

MEAT RECIPES

Crispy Pork Chops

Ingredients (serves 6)

1 ½ lb boneless pork chops
1/3 cup almond flour
¼ cup Parmesan cheese, grated
1 tsp garlic powder
1 tsp paprika
1 tsp Tony Chachere's creole seasoning

Instructions

1. Take a large Ziploc bag and combine all the above ingredients MINUS the pork chops

2. Now add the pork chops, zip the bag shut and shake until the pork chops are fully coated

3. Remove from bag and place into your air fryer basket in a single layer formation.

4. Cook for around 14 minutes. Be sure to check every 5 minutes as cooking time will vary due to the thickness variation in pork chops.

5. Serve!

Carbs: 4g Fiber: 3g Fat: 8g Saturated Fat: 1g Protein: 18g

MARINATED STEAK

Ingredients (serves 2)

2 Butch Box New York Strip Steaks (about 6-8oz each)
1 tablespoon low-sodium soy sauce
1 tsp liquid smoke
1 tablespoon of steak rub
½ tablespoon unsweetened cocoa powder
Salt and pepper

Instructions

1. Using a Ziploc bag, cover the steaks with the soy sauce and liquid smoke

2. Season steak

3. Place in fridge for 2-3 hours

4. Remove and place a couple steaks inside the air fryer basket.

5. Cook for around 5 minutes on 380f for 5 minutes. Cooking times will vary to how you like your steak cooked, so be sure to adjust to this factor by allowing more or less cooking time.

6. Remove steak, drizzle with butter and serve!

Steak rub ingredients: ½ tsp of garlic powder, onion powder, paprika and coriander.

Carbs: 1g Fat: 28g Saturated Fat: 4g Protein: 50g

Buffalo Hot Chicken Wings

Ingredients (serves 6)

16 chicken wing drumettes
2 tsp low-sodium soy sauce
Montreal Grill Mates Chicken Seasoning
Pepper
1 tsp garlic powder
¼ cup Frank's Redhots buffalo wing sauce

Instructions

1. Season the chicken with the Grill Mates seasoning, garlic powder and pepper.

2. Stack the chicken into your air fryer, just make sure not to overcrowd things in there.

3. Spray some cooking oil over the chicken.

4. Set your air fryer to 400 degrees and cook for five mins.

5. Give the pan a shake making sure the chicken is getting cooked evenly.

6. Return the chicken to your air fryer and cook for another 5 mins.

7. Remove from fryer and glaze with hot sauce.

8. Return chicken once more to fryer and cook for 6-12 minutes until the chicken appears well cooked. Make sure to always check chicken isn't pink inside. Serve when desired levels of crispiness are reached!

Carbs: 1g Fiber: 1g Fat: 18g Saturated Fat: 2g Protein: 15g

SICHUAN CUMIN LAMB

Ingredients (serves 4)

1 lb lamb
1.5 tablespoons cumin
½ tsp cayenne
2 tablespoons veg oil
1 tablespoon light soy sauce
1 tablespoon minced garlic
2 red chili peppers
¼ tsp sugar (don't worry, it's such a little amount - it won't hurt)
1 tsp salt
2 scallions
Large handful cilantro

Instructions

1. In a skillet, roast up 2 tablespoons of cumin seeds and a half a tsp of cayenne until fragrant. Give these a grinding with a mortar and pestle once they have cooled.

2. Using a Ziploc bag, marinate the lamb with the above blend and the oil, garlic, red chili peppers, salt, sugar, cumin and soy sauce. You can poke a few holes into the lamb prior to this to allow for a better marinade.

3. Cook the lamb in your air fryer for 10 minutes at a temperature of 360f for ten minutes.

4. Mix in the cilantro (chopped) and scallions (chopped)

5. Serve!

Carbs: 2g Fat: 12g Saturated Fat: 6g Protein: 15g

AIR FRYER NUGGETS

Ingredients **(serves 4)**

1lb free-range boneless, skinless chicken breast
1 tsp sesame oil
Pinch of sea salt
¼ cup coconut flour
½ tsp ground ginger
4 eggs whites
6 tablespoons toasted sesame seeds
Cooking spray

For dip:

2 tablespoons creamy almond butter
1 tablespoon water

2 tsp rice vinegar
4 tsp coconut aminos
1 tsp Sriracha
½ tsp ground ginger
½ tsp monkfruit

Instructions

1. Allow your air fryer to preheat for a good ten mins at 400 degrees

2. Cut your chicken into inch small nuggets. Place them in a bowl and toss with sesame oil and salt

3. Add the chicken, coconut flour and ground ginger into a Ziploc bag and shake until chicken is covered

4. Now put the nuggets into a bowl of egg whites and toss until fully covered

5. Now put the chicken into a Ziploc bag containing the sesame seeds and shake until well covered. Make sure you shake off any excess mixture from the chicken first.

6. Spray your air fryer with your desired cooking spray, add the nuggets and cook for around 6 minutes.

7. Flip the nuggets over as best you can and cook for another 4-6 minutes until the chicken is nice and crisp and of course, no longer pink inside.

8. Mix all the sauce ingredients together in a bowl with a whisk until smooth, then serve with the crisp nuggets

Carbs: 9g Fiber: 5g Fat: 13g Saturated Fat: 4g Protein: 25g

BEEF SATAY

Ingredients (serves 2)

1 lb beef flank steak
1 tablespoon fish sauce
1 tablespoon soy sauce
2 tablespoons oil
1 tablespoon minced garlic
1 tablespoon minced ginger
1 tablespoon sugar
1 tsp Sriracha
1 tsp ground coriander
½ cup chopped cilantro
¼ cup chopped roasted peanuts

Instructions

1. Cut your beef steak into thin strips and place them into a Ziploc bag

2. Now add the fish sauce, oil, ginger, garlic, soy sauce, sugar, Sriracha, coriander and 1/4 cup of cilantro. Give the bag a good shake and marinate in the fridge for 30 minutes.

3. Lay the beef strips side by side in your air fryer and set them to cook for 8 minutes at 400F. Make sure you flip these halfway through!

4. Remove the beef strips, put on a plate, top with remaining cilantro and chopped peanuts.

5. You can serve this with Easy Peanut Sauce for a great taste.

Carbs: 11g Fat: 9g Saturated Fat: 2g Protein: 45g

The Keto Lasagna

Ingredients (serves 4)

1 cup marinara sauce
1 zucchini, sliced
1 cup white onion, diced
1 tsp minced garlic
½ lb mild Italian sausage
½ cup ricotta cheese
½ cup shredded mozzarella
½ cup shredded parmesan
1 egg
½ tsp garlic minced
½ tsp black pepper
½ tsp dried Italian seasoning

Instructions

1. Slice up your zucchini using a mandolin and place it in the bottom of a springform pan. Try and make the zucchini overlap in layers. It's a good idea to spray the pan with oil first.

2. Spread ¼ cup of marinara sauce over the top of your zucchini base until evenly spread.

3. Mix together the sausage, onions and garlic in a large bowl. Now layer the sausage over the zucchini base evenly. Now spread rest of marinara sauce over this.

4. In a bowl, mix together the mozzarella, ricotta and a quarter cup of Parmesan cheese. Spread this mixture on top of the sausage and top with the remaining quarter cup of parmesan cheese.

5. Cover the springform pan with foil and bake for 20 minutes at 350F. Remove foil then cook for 10 more minutes until top is bubbling and golden looking.

6. Let the lasagna sit for 10 mins before removing from the pan, then serve!

Carbs: 8g Fiber: 1g Fat: 30g Saturated Fat: 8g Protein: 15g

BEEF KHEEMA MEATLOAF

Ingredients **(serves 4)**

1 lb ground beef
1 cup onion, diced
2 eggs

¼ cup cilantro, chopped
1 tablespoon minced garlic
1 tablespoon minced ginger
1 tsp salt
2 tsp garam masala
1 tsp turmeric
½ tsp ground cinnamon
1/8 tsp ground cardamom
1 tsp cayenne

Instructions

1. Take a large mixing bowl and combine ALL the ingredients. Mix slowly and gently, but make sure it's well combined eventually.

2. Press the meat mixture 8-inch round cooking pan

3. Cook in your air fryer for 15 mins at a temperature of 360f.

4. Remove, drain excess liquids and serve!

Note: Cut this into 4 pieces and always be sure to check your meat's internal temp by using a meat thermometer.

Carbs: 7g Fiber: 1g Fat: 15g Saturated Fat: 4g Protein: 35g

Ingredients (serves 8)

1 lb ground beef
2 eggs
1 clove garlic, minced
¼ cup onion, chopped
½ cup blanched almond flour
¼ cup sugar-free ketchup
¼ cup coconut flour
½ tsp black pepper
½ tsp salt
1 tablespoon Worcestershire sauce
1 tsp Italian seasoning
½ tsp tarragon

Instructions

1. Combine all ingredients and mix well, making sure everything is combined thoroughly.

2. Shape the meat mixture into 1-inch thick patties. Try and make around 8 of these all the same-ish size.

3. Put patties on a plate and refrigerate them for 10 minutes just so the flour soaks up moisture and makes them firmer.

4. When that time is up, add as many of the patties to your air fryer as you can without cluttering space, and cook for 12 minutes at 360F.

5. Check halfway through, turning if necessary. Do these in batches if they don't all fit in one go.

6. Remove, cover and serve when ready!

Carbs: 6g Fiber: 2g Fat: 18g Saturated Fat: 6g Protein: 12g

PERFECT BACON

Ingredients

Bacon

Instructions

1. Add your bacon to your air fryer in a single layer formation. Fit as many as you can without overlapping.

2. Cook for 10 minutes at 390F

3. Halfway through, flip the bacon over

4. Once 10 minutes are up, check to see how crispy the bacon is and add a couple more minutes on if you want it a little crispier.

5. Serve! From numerous tests with bacon, this temperate and 10-12 minutes has wielded the best results. I've included this in the recipe section as I know bacon can be quite a big part of some people's keto experience!

THE DOUBLE CHEESEBURGER

Ingredients (serves 1)

½ lb ground beef
2 slices of cheddar cheese
Pinch of Sherpa pink Himalayan salt (or preferred salt)
1 pinch fresh ground black pepper
1 pinch onion powder

Instructions

1. Take your beef and form it into two ¼ lb patties.

2. Now lightly season with the pepper, salt and onion powder

3. Cook in your air fryer for 12 minutes at a temperature of 370F for 12 minutes.

4. Flip the burgers half way through and continue to cook.

5. Once the 12 minutes are up, add the cheese on top of your burgers, shut the drawer and give it a quick minute blast to melt the cheese.

6. These burgers go great with low-carb buns. Take a look at the snacks and appetizers section of this book for a keto-friendly bun recipe!

Carbs: 1g Fat: 48g Saturated Fat: 9g Protein: 35g

Spicy Lamb Sirloin Steak

Ingredients (serves 4)

1 lb boneless lamb sirloin steaks
4 slices ginger
5 garlic cloves
½ onion
1 tsp ground fennel
1 tsp garam masala
1 tsp ground cinnamon
½ tsp cayenne
1 tsp salt
½ tsp ground cardamom

Instructions

1. In a blender, pulse and blend ALL the ingredients EXCEPT for the lamb steaks. Make sure ingredients are well blended – should take 3 or 4 mins.

2. Now, in a large bowl, marinate the lamb in the above mixture.

3. Rest the mixture for 30 mins in the refrigerator.

4. Remove when time is up and add them to your air fryer in a single layer formation.

5. Cook for 15 mins at a temperate of 330F, flipping halfway through cooking time.

6. As per usual, always use a meat thermometer to check the temperature (150F for medium well) before serving!

Carbs: 2g Fiber: 1g Fat: 10g Saturated Fat: 2g Protein: 25g

KOREAN GRILLED PORK

Ingredients (serves 4)

1 lb boneless pork shoulder
1 onion
2 tablespoons Korean red pepper paste
1 tablespoon minced garlic
1 tablespoon minced ginger
1 tablespoon rice wine
1 tablespoon soy sauce
1 tablespoon sesame oil
1 tsp sugar
¼ tsp cayenne pepper
1 tablespoon sesame seeds
¼ cup green onions

Instructions

1. Cut the pork shoulder into half inch thick slices. Chop your green onions too.

2. Mix together the onion, red pepper paste, ginger, cayenne, soy sauce, rice wine, sesame oil, cayenne, sugar, garlic and pork.

3. Allow this mixture to marinate in the fridge for 30 mins.

4. When finished, at the pork and onions into your air fryer basket. Get rid of any of the excess marinade or save it for other recipes.

5. Cook for 15 minutes at a temperate of 400F, flipping half way.

6. Check with meat thermometer and serve!

Carbs: 1g Fat: 12g Saturated Fat: 1g Protein: 25g

SNACKS AND APPETIZERS

CAULIFLOWER WINGS

Ingredients **(serves 4)**

3 tablespoons low-carb hot sauce
1 tablespoon avocado oil
1 tablespoon almond flour
Salt
1 medium sized cauliflower head, chopped

Instructions

1. In a large bowl, mix together the almond flour, avocado oil, salt and hot sauce.

2. Now add the cauliflower and coat well

3. Cook HALF the cauliflower batch in your air fryer for 14-17 mins, turning halfway through

4. Remove and cook the second batch for 12-15 minutes

5. Serve!

Carbs: 3g Fat: 10g Saturated Fat: 2g Protein: 2g

CRISPY KALE CHIPS

Ingredients (serves 4)

4 cups kale
½ tsp salt
1 tablespoon olive oil

Instructions

1. Mix together the kale, salt and oil. Make sure that all the ribs are removed from the kale first – the kale won't cook into a crispy state otherwise.

2. Cook in the air fryer for 5 minutes at 370F

3. Shake half way through to make sure the kale is getting cooked all over

4. Transfer to a suitable bowl and serve!

Carbs: 10g Fiber: 1g Fat: 7g Saturated Fat: 1g Protein: 2g

QUICK SUMMER ZUCCHINI

Ingredients (serves 4)

1 lb zucchini sliced into 'circles'
1 tsp Kosher salt
½ tsp black pepper
1 tsp garlic powder
2 tablespoon extra-virgin olive oil

Instructions

1. Slice the zucchini into rounds to form ¼ inch thick circle-like shapes

2. Now, in a smallish bowl, combine the seasonings and olive oil. Mix well.

3. Add the zucchini slices into the above mixture and combine thoroughly.

4. Add the zucchini to your air fryer basket and cook for around 35 minutes on 400F. Be sure to toss every ten minutes to ensure all the slices are evenly cooked.

5. Serve when desired level of browning has occurred.

Carbs: 10g Fiber: 4.5g Fat: 2.8g Saturated Fat: 1g Protein: 5g

Cheesy Pickles

Ingredients (serves 2-4)

2 cups dill pickles, sliced
1 egg
1 cup low-carb bread crumbs
½ cup parmesan
Seasoning to taste

Instructions

1. Dry your sliced pickles out on a couple pieces of paper towel. Try and remove as much liquid as possible.

2. You need 3 bowls for these next steps.

3. In the first bowl, add your egg and a tsp of water. Add the breadcrumbs to the second bowl (with any seasonings), and in the third bowl, your cheese.

4. Take a fork and 'drag' the pickles one by one through each of the bowls until fully coated. Make sure you use shallow bowls to avoid any mess.

5. Add as many as you can to your air fryer basket, until the bottom is full, and you can no longer single layer them. SINGLE LAYER – do not stack.

6. You probably won't be able to fit all in one go, so cook these in batches.

7. Bake at 400F for 5 minutes, turn and bake for a further 4-5 minutes until crisp. Serve when all are completed!

Carbs: 1g Fiber: 1g Fat: 15g Saturated Fat: 0g Protein: 4g

KETO FRIENDLY SCOTCH EGGS

Ingredients (serves 4)

1 lb bulk pork sausage
2 tablespoons fresh parsley, chopped
1 tablespoon fresh chives, chopped
1/8 tsp grated nutmeg
1/8 tsp salt
1/8 tsp ground black pepper
4 eggs, peeled – hard-cooked
2 tsp coarse ground mustard
1 cup parmesan cheese, shredded

Instructions

1. Combine the sausage, chives, mustard, salt, nutmeg and black pepper in a large bowl.

2. Form the mixture into 4 patties of an equal size

3. Shape each of the patties around the hard-cooked eggs until completely covered in a ball like shape.

4. Now roll each of the eggs over the parmesan cheese until covered entirely. You want to make sure that the cheese is compact on the sausage mixture.

5. Set the eggs into your air fryer, give them a small spray with veg oil and cook at 400F for 15 mins. Turn eggs halfway through and spray with oil again.

6. Remove carefully and serve with the ground mustard!

Carbs: 3g Fat: 20g Saturated Fat: 2g Protein: 30g

BACON WRAPPED SPROUTS

Ingredients **(serves 4)**

½ lb brussels sprouts
Canola oil spray
1 tsp lemon pepper seasoning
5 slices centre cut bacon

Instructions

1. Cut your sprouts into halves and add them to a medium sized bowl. Spray very lightly with oil until coated

2. Add the lemon pepper seasoning and toss until sprouts are evenly covered

3. Stack all 5 slices of bacon and cut them into strips by halving them lengthwise and then widthwise so that each piece now becomes 4 pieces.

4. Wrap the sprouts in the bacon. One quarter piece of bacon per sprout.

5. Place them into your air fryer, with the 'seam' side facing down. Cook on 400F for 10-15 minutes, checking regularly until desired outcome is reached.

6. Serve and enjoy!

Carbs: 1g Fat: 18g Saturated Fat: 5g Protein: 6g

AIR FRIED ASPARAGUS

***Ingredients* (serves 4)**

½ bunch of asparagus
Avocado oil
Black pepper
Himalayan salt
Instructions

1. Trim the asparagus. Take off the bottom 2 inches of each spear.

2. Place each spear into your air fryer and spritz lightly with your avocado oil.

3. Sprinkle on the salt and pepper

4. Bake for 10 mins at 400F

5. Serve!

Carbs: 1g Fiber: 1g Fat: 1g Saturated Fat: 0g Protein: 2g

KETO FRIENDLY BURGER BUN

Ok, so – this isn't an air fryer recipe, BUT, I've had a lot of requests for a simple low-carb bun recipe that can be used when making beef and chicken burgers. So, here it is!

Ingredients

2 cups mozzarella
4 oz cream cheese
3 large eggs
3 cups almond flour
2 tsp baking powder
4 tablespoons butter
1 tsp kosher salt
Dried parsley
Sesame seeds

Instructions

1. Preheat oven to 400 degrees.

2. Use parchment paper to line a baking sheet.

3. Melt together the cream cheese and mozzarella in an appropriate bowl.

4. Now add the eggs, stir to combine. Slowly add the almond flour, salt and baking powder. Stir again.

5. Form this mixture into 6 balls, then flatten each onto the baking sheet you prepared earlier.

6. Give each a brush with some butter. Sprinkle some sesame seeds and parsley over the top too, if you like.

7. Bake for around 10-13 minutes or until golden!

Mozzarella Sticks

Ingredients (serves 4)

6 pieces string cheese
1 large egg
¼ cup parmesan cheese
¼ cup almond flour
1 tablespoon coconut flour
½ tsp garlic powder
½ tsp Kosher salt
1 tsp Italian seasoning

Instructions

1. Take the string cheese and cut in half along the length of each piece.

2. Using a Ziploc bag, mix together the Parmesan cheese, almond flour, coconut flour, garlic powder, Italian seasoning and salt.

3. Mix the large egg into a bowl and then dip each cheese string in until fully covered.

4. Now add each cheese string to the Ziploc bag in step 2 and shake until all pieces are fully coated.

5. Freeze for one hour.

6. When ready, place into air fryer and cook for 5 minutes at a temperature of 400F.

7. Turn each piece halfway through to ensure they are evenly cooked. They should turn nice and brown on all sides! Serve!

Carbs: 2g Fat: 5g Saturated Fat: 1g Protein: 4g

TOMATILLO SALSA

Ingredients (serves 4)

12 tomatillos
2 serrano peppers, stems removed
1 cup cilantro, chopped
1 tablespoon minced garlic
1 tsp salt

Instructions

1. Wash the tomatillos and remove husks.

2. Take a heatproof pan, one that fits your air fryer and add the peppers, whole tomatillos and garlic.

3. Place pan in air fryer and cook for 15 mins at a temperature of 305F.

4. When finished, pour mixture into blender and puree until smooth.

5. Pour into serving dish and add salt and chopped cilantro.

Carbs: 17g Fat: 6g Protein: 3g

SHISHITO PEPPERS

Ingredients (serves 4)

1 6oz bag Shishito peppers
Salt and pepper
½ tablespoon avocado oil
1/3 cup Asiago cheese
Limes

Instructions

1. Give the peppers a rinse, then pat them dry with paper towels. Now place them into a bowl with the avocado oil, salt and pepper.

2. Toss until fully covered.

3. Place into your air fryer basket and cook for 10 mins at a temperate of 350F.

4. Remove, drizzle with lime cheese and top with the cheese.

5. Serve!

Carbs: 1g Fat: 4g Protein: 3g

ROASTED OKRA

Ingredients **(serves 1)**

½ lb okra
1 tsp olive oil
¼ tsp salt
1/8 tsp ground black pepper

Instructions

1. Trim the ends and slice the pods of your okra.

2. In a medium sized bowl, mix together the okra, salt, pepper and olive oil. Stir gently until fully combined

3. Layer okra in a single layer formation in your air fryer basket and cook for 7 minutes at a temperate of 350F.

4. Toss okra then cook for another 5 mins.

5. Toss once more then cook for another minute and then serve! Simple but truly delicious snack!

Carbs: 4g Fiber: 2g Fat: 2g Protein: 2g

KETO FRIES

Ingredients (serves 4)

1 medium sized jicama
½ tsp garlic powder
1 tsp smoked paprika
2 tablespoons olive oil
Salt and pepper to taste

Instructions

1. Cut the jicama into fry-like shapes, whatever size you prefer them. I personally prefer them thin.

2. Now, in a large bowl, combine the jicama, smoked paprika, olive oil, garlic powder and a little salt and pepper. Combine thoroughly.

3. Set your air fryer to 400F and cook the fries for 15 minutes. Give the basket a shake every 5 minutes to make sure the chips are being fried evenly.

4. Serve!

Carbs: 10g Fiber: 4g Fat: 8g Protein: 1g

SEAFOOD RECIPES

SHRIMP SCAMPI

Ingredients (serves 4)

1 lb defrosted shrimp (around 25 count)

4 tablespoons butter
1 tablespoon minced garlic
1 tablespoon lemon juice
2 tsp red pepper flakes
1 tablespoon chives, chopped
1 tablespoon minced basil leaves
2 tablespoons chicken stock

Instructions

1. Use a 6x3 metal pan for this recipe. Place it into your air fryer and set the temperature to 330F and allow it to heat while you prepare the rest of your food.

2. Add the red pepper flakes, garlic and butter to the now hot pan.

3. Cook this for a couple minutes, stirring occasionally until melted.

4. Now open your fryer and add the rest of the ingredients. Stir.

5. Cook for 5 minutes, stirring occasionally.

6. Remove from fryer and set to one side to rest for 1 minute. The residual heat will finish the meal off nicely.

7. Stir and serve with chopped basil leaves!

Carbs: 1g Fiber: 1g Fat: 15g Saturated Fat: 7g Protein: 23g

TOMATO BASIL SCALLOPS

Ingredients **(serves 2)**

8 jumbo sea scallops
¾ cup heavy whipping cream
1 tablespoon tomato paste
1 tsp minced garlic
1 tablespoon fresh basil, chopped
½ tsp salt
½ tsp pepper
12 oz pack of spinach

Instructions

1. Take a 7-inch heatproof pan, spray it with oil lightly and add the spinach across the bottom of it in a single layer.

2. Lightly spray each side of all your scallops. Sprinkle a little bit of salt and pepper on them, then add them to the pan over the top of the spinach.

3. Now, in a medium sized bowl, mix up the tomato paste, heavy whipping cream, garlic, basil, salt and pepper. Pour this mixture over your scallops.

4. Add to your air fryer and cook at 350F for ten mins or until scallops appear to be fully cooked.

5. Serve!

Carbs: 6g Fat: 33g Saturated Fat: 20g Protein: 9g

FISH EN PAPILLOTE

Ingredients **(serves 2)**

2 5oz cod fillets

½ cup julienned fennel bulbs
½ cup julienned carrots
2 sprigs tarragon
½ cup red peppers, sliced
2 pats melted butter
1 tablespoon salt
1 tablespoon lemon juice
1 tablespoon oil
½ teaspoon pepper

Instructions

1. Combine melted butter, ½ tsp salt, lemon juice and tarragon in a medium sized bowl. Mix until creamy.

2. Now add the julienned vegs and mix well.

3. Take some parchment paper and cut two squares from it that are large enough to hold the fish and veg

4. Lay the fillets down on the parchment paper, one on each square.

5. Top each of the cod fillets with half of your veg mix.

6. Fold the parchment paper of the fish and veg, crimping the sides so it holds the fish, veg and sauce firmly.

7. Add these to your air fryer and cook for 15 mins at 350F. Remove then serve!

Carbs: 9g Fiber: 2g Fat: 13g Saturated Fat: 2g Protein: 20g

Spicy Crab Dip

Ingredients (serves 4)

1 cooked crab
2 cups grated jalapeno jack cheese
¼ cup mayonnaise
2 tablespoons low-carb hot sauce
½ cup scallions
½ tsp salt
1 tsp pepper
2 tablespoons parsley, chopped
2 tablespoons lemon juice

Instructions

1. Mix together the crab, cheese, mayo, scallion, hot sauce, salt and pepper in a 6-inch heatproof pan.

2. Add the pan to your air fryer and cook for 7 mins at 400F until completely melted.

3. Remove, mix in the parsley and lemon juice.

4. Serve nice and hot!

Carbs: 2g Fat: 28g Saturated Fat: 12g Protein: 21g

Tomato Mayonnaise Shrimp

Ingredients (serves 4)

1 lb large 21-25 count peeled, tail-on shrimp
1 tablespoon sugar-free ketchup
3 tablespoons mayonnaise
1 tablespoon minced garlic
½ tsp smoked paprika
1 tsp sriracha
½ tsp salt
½ cup green onions, chopped

Instructions

1. Mix together the salt, paprika, ketchup, sriracha, garlic and mayo in a large or medium sized bowl.

2. Now add in the shrimp and toss until shrimp is completely coated.

3. Place the shrimp into a pre-greased basket in your air fryer.

4. Cook for 8 mins at 325F. Toss the shrimps half way through, making sure to spray with oil again.

5. Remove and serve with chopped green onions!

Carbs: 2g Fat: 8g Saturated Fat: 2g Protein: 20g

Rosemary Grilled Prawns

Ingredients (serves 4)

8 large sized prawns
4 garlic cloves, minced
½ tablespoon butter
1 sprig rosemary leaves, chopped
Salt and black pepper
8 slices green capsicum

Instructions

1. In a medium sized bowl, add the prawns with all seasoning ingredients and allow to marinate for one hour.

2. Preheat your air fryer to 355F.

3. Skewer 2 prawns and 2 capsicums per skewer.

4. Grill the prawns for around 5 or 6 mins, then increase the temperate to 395F and grill for a further minute.

5. Serve when all 4 sets of prawn have been cooked!

Carbs: 3g Fiber: 1g Fat: 18g Saturated Fat: 7g Protein: 25g

TUNA PATTIES

Ingredients (serves 2)

2 can tuna, water packed
1.5 tablespoons mayonnaise
1.5 tablespoons almond flour
1 tsp garlic powder

1 tsp dried dill
½ tsp onion powder
Pinch of salt and pepper
Juice of half a lemon

Instructions

1. In a large bowl, combine all the ingredients and mix slowly but thoroughly.

2. Form patty shapes with resulting mixture. You should be able to make 4 decent size patties. If the mixture isn't dry enough to make a solid patty, then just add a little more almond flour until it is.

3. Add your patties in a single-layer formation to your air fryer and cook for 10 mins at 400F. You can cook for a few minutes longer if you want them a little crispier.

4. Remove and serve!

Note: You can always double the ingredients of my recipes to make even more!

Carbs: 10g Fat: 28g Saturated Fat: 8g Protein: 35g

CHILI LIME SALMON

Ingredients (serves 2)

1 lb Alaska king salmon, fresh
¼ tsp pepper
½ tsp chili powder
¼ tsp salt

2 whole limes
Fresh parsley for garnishing

Instructions

1. Take your salmon and season it with salt, pepper and chili powder.

2. Slice a lime and place it on the salmon

3. Add the salmon to your air fryer and cook for around 9 minutes at a temperature of 375F.

4. You should use a meat thermometer to check the fish has reached a temp of 145 degrees.

5. Squeeze juice from the remaining lime onto the salmon after you've removed it from your air fryer.

6. Garnish with chopped fresh parsley and serve!

Carbs: 1g Fat: 18g Saturated Fat: 2g Protein: 35g

CAJUN SHRIMP

Ingredients (serves 2)

½ lb shrimp, deveined and peeled
½ tsp old bay seasoning
¼ tsp smoked paprika
¾ tsp cayenne pepper
Pinch of salt
1 tablespoon olive oil

Instructions

1. Make sure that your shrimp are completely peeled and deveined before starting.

2. Take a large mixing bowl and add all the ingredients.

3. Slowly coat the shrimp by tossing it around in the bowl. Make sure it's completely covered.

4. Set your air fryer to 390F and cook the shrimp for 6 minutes.

5. You can turn these half way through cooking time and add additional time if needed.

6. Serve!

Carbs: 0.6g Fat: 9g Saturated Fat: 2g Protein: 10g

CRAB CAKES

Ingredients (serves 4)

1 cup gluten-free breadcrumbs (have found this to be best for this recipe)
¼ cup mayonnaise
12 ounces crab meat
2 green onions, chopped
1 egg
1 tablespoon lemon juice
1 tsp old bay seasoning
1 tsp red pepper flakes

Instructions

1. In a large bowl, mix together half a cup of the bread crumbs, green onion and mayonnaise.

2. Now add the crab meat, egg, lemon juice and seasonings. Combine until thoroughly mixed.

3. You should now be able to make around 8 small cakes from this mixture.

4. Dip each cake into the remaining breadcrumbs.

5. Set your air fryer to 400F and cook for 7 minutes. Flip each cake over and cook for a further 5-7 minutes. Add additional time if needed. If the cakes don't fit in one go, cook them in batches.

6. Remove and serve!

Carbs: 1g Fat: 12g Saturated Fat: 2g Protein: 15g

CAJUN SALMON

Ingredients (serves 1-2)

1 piece fresh salmon fillet
Cajun seasoning
Juice from quarter of lemon

Instructions

1. Preheat air fryer to 355F.

2. Pat your salmon dry and on a plate sprinkle the Cajun over the entirety of the salmon in a thin layer.

3. If your macronutrients allow it, you can at this point sprinkle a tiny amount of sugar over the sides also, to add some sweetness.

4. Cook in air fryer grill for 7 minutes with the skin side facing up.

5. Serve directly after cooking and add a squeeze of lemon!

Carbs: 1g Fat: 35g Saturated Fat: 5g Protein: 40g

JALAPENO POPPERS

Ingredients **(serves 4)**

5 medium jalapenos
2 eggs
8 oz cream cheese
Coconut oil spray
7 oz canned salmon
½ tsp red pepper flakes
2 slices cooked bacon
1 oz Whisps (any flavor)
2 oz pork rinds

Instructions

1. Blender together the Whisps and pork rinds. Blend until they form an almost dust-like texture. Transfer to a bowl and set aside for now.

2. Now cut the jalapenos lengthwise and core center. Set aside.

3. In a large bowl, add warmed cream cheese (microwave for a minute) and canned salmon. Sprinkle in red pepper flakes and mix until fully combined.

4. Chop up the slices of cooked bacon, add to above mixture and mix.

5. Stuff the jalapenos with the mixture and set aside for a moment.

6. Take two eggs and whisk them in a bowl. Now cover each of the jalapenos with the egg mixture first and then the Whisps mixture from step 1 until fully covered.

7. Place some parchment paper into your air fryer, add peppers (do these in batches depending on how many fit) and cook for 320F for 15 mins.

8. Remove and spray lightly with coconut oil before returning to the air fryer. Cook until it looks nicely crisped!

9. Serve!

Carbs: 4g Fiber: 1g Fat: 13g Protein: 15g

Vegetarian Recipes

Herb and Cheese Frittata

Ingredients (serves 4)

4 eggs
1/3 cup cheddar cheese, shredded
½ cup 'half and half'
2 tablespoons green scallions, chopped
2 tablespoons cilantro, chopped
½ tsp ground pepper
½ tsp salt

Instructions

1. Grease up an oven-safe 6-inch pan, making sure it's one that fits your air fryer.

2. Mix together the eggs and 'half-and-half'. Beat well.

3. Now stir in all the remaining ingredients then add to your 6-inch pan.

4. Place your 6-inch pan into your air fryer and cook for 15 minutes at a temperate of 330F

5. Carefully remove when time is up. Frittata should be set nicely. Give additional time if it isn't quite to your liking.

6. Serve!

Carbs: 2g Fat: 10g Saturated Fat: 5g Protein: 8g

SPICY CAULIFLOWER STIR-FRY

Ingredients (serves 4)

1 head cauliflower
¾ cup onion, thinly sliced
5 cloves garlic, sliced
1 tablespoon rice vinegar
1 ½ tablespoons tamari
½ tsp coconut sugar
1 tablespoon Sriracha
2 scallions

Instructions

1. Cut cauliflower head into florets then add to air fryer.

2. Cook for 10 mins at a temperate of 350F.

3. Now add onion and cook for a further 10 mins.

4. Add garlic, stir, cook for another 5 mins.

5. In a small bowl, mix together the rice vinegar, Sriracha, soy sauce, coconut sugar and a pinch of salt and pepper.

6. When cauliflower is finished cooking, add the above mixture to the cauliflower in your air fryer and cook for 5 more mins.

7. Serve with scallions sprinkled over!

Carbs: 11g Fiber: 3g Fat: 4g Protein: 3g

KETO PIZZA

Ingredients (serves 4)

¾ cup fine almond flour
1 whole egg
Italian seasoning
Pepper flakes
Garlic
1.5 cups mozzarella cheese
2 tablespoon ricotta cheese

Instructions

1. In a microwaveable bowl, add the mozzarella cheese and ricotta cheese. Microwave for 1 minute and 20 seconds. If the mixture is still a bit stringy, you can microwave for a little longer.

2. Now add the almond flour, egg, Italian seasoning, pepper flakes and garlic. Mix well.

3. Form this mixture into a ball, then flatten using a rolling pin on some parchment paper.

4. Use a springform pan to cut the shape out of as many pizzas as you can. If you don't have one, find something that allows you to cut the dough into a circular shape.

5. Place your springform pan into your air fryer (one at a time) and cook for 6 minutes at 320F.

6. Cooking time will vary depending on your springform pan size so please monitor your cooking.

7. You can, after removing the pizza, add whatever toppings you desire and then give them another blast in the air fryer before serving!

Carbs: 9g Fat: 20g Saturated Fat: 6g Protein: 3g

KETO AIR FRYER TOAST

Ingredients **(serves 4)**

Section 1:

3 tablespoons almond flour
1 egg
1 tablespoon coconut oil
½ tsp baking powder
Pinch of salt

Section 2:

Heavy whipping cream
Splenda
Cinnamon
1 egg

Instructions

1. Take a mug of your choice, doesn't matter too much on the size as long as it's not tiny.

2. Combine all ingredients into the mug and stir until a thick mixture has formed at the bottom.

3. Microwave mug and mixture for 90 seconds.

4. Remove and cut mixture into 3 or 4 slices.

5. Splash a small amount of heavy whipping cream into a bowl along with another egg, a dash of cinnamon and half a teaspoon of Splenda. Whisk mixture until combined.

6. Egg wash each of the slices, fully covering each! Add all of the slices to your air fryer basket and cook for 4 minutes at a temperature of 350F.

7. Keep an eye on the slices as you may want to add more time. Serve when ready!

Carbs: 10g Fat: 13g Saturated Fat: 2g Protein: 5g

Cauliflower Pizza Crust

Ingredients (serves 4)

½ pack organic riced cauliflower, steamed
2 eggs
1 cup mozzarella
1 tablespoon garlic powder
¼ cup psyllium powder

Instructions

1. Take your rice cauliflower and steam it in your microwave for around 4 minutes. It should be nice and tender when taken out.

2. Use a strainer to push out as much water as you can from the cauliflower rice. You can use a spoon to push on it.

3. Set your air fryer to 400F and preheat it for 5 mins.

4. Now, in a medium sized bowl, add all the ingredients except for the psyllium powder and mix until it looks dry. Add the psyllium as you are mixing (before it gets dry).

5. Place the dough into the air fryer and flatten it out to whatever thickness you'd like.

6. Cook for 10-15 mins. Pizza crust should be a nice golden-brown color before removing and serving!

8. Put whatever topping you like on, then add it back to the air fryer until cheese melts on top.

9. Serve!

Carbs: 3g Fiber: 1g Fat: 11g Saturated Fat: 4g Protein: 2g

Cheesy Bagels

Ingredients (serves 6)

1 ¼ cup almond flour
½ cup coconut flour
1 tablespoon baking powder
2 ½ cups shredded mozzarella
2 oz softened cream cheese
2 large eggs
1 egg, beaten in a separate bowl

Instructions

1. In a small bowl, mix together the coconut flour, almond flour and baking powder.

2. In a separate bowl, beat together the two large eggs.

3. Now microwave the mozzarella and cream cheese in a suitable bowl for around 1 minute. Remove and stir, then place back into microwave for a further minute. Remove and stir again.

4. Now add the flour mixture from step 1 and stir slowly until combined.

5. Add the beaten eggs from step 2 and knead the dough with your hands until a ball is formed.

6. Separate the dough into 6 pieces, roll each piece out into a snake-like shape, and then bring the ends together to form the bagel shape. Pinch the ends on all 6 to make sure they are well attached.

7. If you wish to add toppings, then you can brush the remaining egg over the top and bottom of each bagel and then add your toppings.

8. Preheat your fryer to 370F for 8 minutes. Place parchment paper into basket and spray with some oil.

9. Now add as many bagels as you can without the air fryer getting crowed, this is probably going to be about 3 at a time.

10. Cook for 4 mins on each side. Repeat this for all batches.

11. Serve!

Carbs: 6g Fiber: 3g Fat: 18g Protein: 10g

Cauliflower Parmesan Cups

Ingredients **(serves 4)**

2 cups cauliflower florets
1 egg

½ cup parmesan, grated
½ tsp garlic powder
½ tsp Italian seasoning
½ tsp crushed black pepper
¼ cup olive oil
1 cup prepared meat sauce
½ cup mozzarella, shredded

Instructions

1. Blend the cauliflower into a rice-like texture in a food blender.

2. Now add in the grated parmesan, Italian seasoning, garlic powder, egg, black pepper and olive oil. Blend until mixture is well combined.

3. Take some mini tartlet pans and grease them lightly. Now add a tablespoon of the mixture into each tartlet pan. The numbers may vary depending on the size of your pans, just fill up as many as you can.

4. Using your fingers, press the mixture down into the pans and up the sides to form a cup-like shape with the mixture.

5. Place your pans into the air fryer and cook for 10 mins at a temperate of 350F. You might need to cook these in batches if all the pans don't fit in one go.

6. Remove from air fryer and add 2 teaspoons of meat sauce to each cup and top with shredded mozzarella.

7. Return to air fryer and cook for another 5 mins. Remove and serve!

Carbs: 4g Fat: 18g Saturated Fat: 6g Protein: 4g

DESSERT RECIPES

FLOURLESS BROWNIES

Ingredients **(serves 14 pieces)**

6 tablespoons coconut oil
225 grams 100% baking chocolate
¾ cup granulated sweetener of choice
2 large eggs
3 tablespoons arrowroot powder
2 tablespoon unsweetened cocoa powder
¼ cup sugar-free chocolate chips

Instructions

1. Melt the coconut oil and baking chocolate into a microwaveable bowl and stir until smooth.

2. Line a brownie pan (one that fits your instant pot) with parchment paper and set to one side for now.

3. Now add the rest of the ingredients to the mixture in step 1 and mix well.

4. Now fill as much of your brownie pan as possible with the mixture. Use two batches if your pan isn't big enough.

5. Place in air fryer and cook for 30 minutes at temperate of 350F. Be sure to keep checking up on your brownies as there is some room for error in this recipe.

6. Serve!

Carbs: 10g Fiber: 1g Fat: 15g Saturated Fat: 2g Protein: 3g

ALMOND FLOUR DONUTS

Ingredients (serves 12 donuts)

1 cup almond flour
4 eggs
¼ sugar substitute (I used erythritol)
¼ tsp salt
¼ tsp baking powder
¼ tsp cinnamon
1 tsp vanilla extract

Instructions

1. In a large bowl, whisk together the eggs, sugar substitute and vanilla extract.

2. Now add the baking powder, almond flour, cinnamon and salt. Whisk again until the mixture is thick but smooth.

3. If you have a donut mold, use that to shape your donuts. If not, you can simply roll the dough into 12 small balls

4. Place into air fryer basket and cook for 15 mins at a temperature of 280F.

5. Keep an eye on how these are doing, they made need less time, they may need more.

6. Serve!

Carbs: 6g Fiber: 1g Fat: 5g Protein: 6g

LAVA CAKE

Ingredients (serves 2)

1 egg
2 tablespoons water
2 tablespoons cocoa powder, unsweetened
2 tablespoons erythritol
1/8 tsp Stevia
1 tablespoon golden flaxmeal
1 tablespoon coconut oil
½ tsp baking powder
Dash of vanilla
Pinch of Himalayan salt

Instructions

1. Whisk together all the ingredients in a Pyrex glass dish. Ideally, a two-cup sized Pyrex would be best. If you have ramekins that can do the job, then use them – just make sure there is enough room to whisk it.

2. Preheat air fryer to 350F.

3. Place your Pyrex/ramekin into the air fryer just 1 minute after preheating.

4. Bake the mixture for 8-10 minutes at a temperate of 350F.

5. Remove and serve! (give it a minute to cool, it might be quite hot).

Carbs: 4g Fiber: 1g Fat: 13g Protein: 8g

CHOCOLATE AVOCADO PUDDING

Ingredients

Ok, so this isn't an air fryer recipe. However, it is totally keto and SO good that I know you'll just love it. It's simple, healthy, keto friendly and super delicious!

3 avocados (small ones)
½ cup erythritol
½ cup almond milk or coconut milk
½ cup Stevia or prefer sweetener
2 tablespoons raw cacao

¾ tsp vanilla
Pinch of salt

Instructions

1. Put your avocados into a blender (peeled and stone removed obviously)

2. Now add the rest of the ingredients and blend slow to begin with. Once the ingredients have blended a little, turn the blender up and blend into a smooth mixture.

3. That's it – serve!

Carbs: 10g Fiber: 6g Fat: 15g Protein: 3g

CREAM CHEESE COOKIES

Ingredients (serves 9 pieces)

½ cup cream cheese
½ cup erythritol
2 cups almond flour
¼ cup butter
1 egg
Pinch of salt

Instructions

1. Use a hand blender to mix together the erythritol, butter and cream cheese. Blend until creamy.

2. Now add the egg and salt to the mixture. Start adding the almond flour slowly and blend until mixture is soft and runny.

3. Now spoon the mixture into a suitably sized pan, making sure it's one that fits your air fryer. You might need to bake the cookies in batches if you can't fit 9 in at once. Make sure your baking tray is lined with parchment paper.

4. Bake for 12-15 minutes at a temperate of 325F. Keep an eye on the cookies as you cook them.

5. Leave to cool, then serve!

Carbs: 7g Fat: 5g Protein: 6g

Part 2

INTRODUCTION

Welcome to "Easy Ketogenic Air Fryer Cookbook For Beginners". If you are new to the air fryer, here's what you should know: An air fryer is a countertop kitchen appliance promising crispy, fried to perfection foods that are much healthier. It uses superheated airflow above and around food to convert tiny amounts of moisture into mist. The extra-hot cooking chamber lets dry heat penetrate the food from the outside in, yielding the familiar crispy texture food gets with a bath in the deep fryer.

Most air fryers don't require oil for the machine to work, though a couple of teaspoons will improve the texture and flavor of air-fried eats. While it's possible to enjoy air-fried food with no oil, the beauty of the air fryer is that it only needs such a small amount.

The little bit of oil you do add help everything brown, caramelize and get extra crispy and delicious. And compared to the amount of oil and calories in deep-fried foods, the amount you'll use in the air fryer is practically nothing.

You can cook just about anything from fish, meats, veggie dishes, to desserts, appetizers and side dishes in an air fryer.

This cookbook invites you to discover 100 healthy and delicious keto meals that you can make in an air fryer. Choose from 8 categories including quick and easy breakfasts or snacks, delicious meat, fish or poultry recipes and even healthy keto desserts. Enjoy!

NUTRITIOUS SNACKS AND APPETIZERS

1. Hazelnut Crusted Cheddar Sticks

Full-flavored sticks of cheddar in a crisp savory hazelnut crust. This recipe brings your typical cheese sticks to a whole new level.

DETAILS:

- Preparation Time: 10 minutes
- Cooking Time: 8 min
- Serves: 8

NUTRITIONAL VALUES:

- Kcal per serve: 263
- Fat: 22 g. (76%)
- Protein: 13 g. (20%)
- Carbs: 3 g. (4%)

INGREDIENTS:

- 300 grams Cheddar Cheese, cut into sticks
- 100 grams Hazelnuts, ground
- 2 Eggs, beaten
- ½ tsp Italian Herb Seasoning

PREPARATION:

Mix together ground hazelnuts and Italian seasoning.

Dip cheese sticks in egg then coat in hazelnut mixture.

Coat the fryer basket with non-stick spray.

Arrange cheese sticks in the frying basket.

Cook for 8 minutes at 390F flipping halfway through the cooking time.

2. SAUSAGE AND CREAM CHEESE STUFFED MUSHROOMS

Smoky minced chorizo and rich cream cheese give life to this roasted mushroom appetizer. Perfect bite-sized keto goodness!

DETAILS:

- Preparation Time: 24 hours
- Cooking Time: 20 min
- Serves: 6

NUTRITIONAL VALUES:

- Kcal per serve: 259
- Fat: 22 g. (77%)
- Protein: 11 g. (18%)
- Carbs: 3 g. (5%)

INGREDIENTS:

- 250 grams Brown Mushrooms
- 200 grams Minced Chorizo
- 200 grams Cream Cheese
- 1 tbsp Fresh Parsley, minced

PREPARATION:

Blend together minced chorizo, cream cheese, and fresh parsley.

Stuff the mixture into the mushrooms.

Coat the fryer basket with non-stick spray.

Arrange stuffed mushrooms in the frying basket.

Cook for 10 minutes at 380F.

3. MASALA AND CHEESE CAULIFLOWER TOTS

Looking for a low-carb alternative to those highly addictive tater tots? You just may find these Masala-spiked cauliflower nibblers even better you'd never look back to that carb-rich potato favorite.

DETAILS:

- Preparation Time: 5 min
- Cooking Time: 8 min
- Serves: 4

NUTRITIONAL VALUES:

- Kcal per serve: 148
- Fat: 12 g. (73%)

- Protein: 5 g. (13%)
- Carbs: 5 g. (14%)

INGREDIENTS:

- 300 grams Cauliflower, cut into florets
- ½ cup grated Parmesan
- 1 tsp garam Masala
- 3 tbsp Butter, melted

PREPARATION:

Combine all ingredients in a resealable bag. Shake well to coat evenly.

Coat the fryer basket with non-stick spray.

Arrange cauliflower pieces in the frying basket.

Cook for 8 minutes at 380F.

4. Air Fryer Jalapeno Poppers

Hot jalapeno peppers stuffed with gooey cheese and crisp bacon bits. Yes, the party-favorite can be done in the air fryer too!

DETAILS:

- Preparation Time: 15 min
- Cooking Time: 5 min
- Serves: 4

NUTRITIONAL VALUES:

- Kcal per serve: 218
- Fat: 18 g. (77%)
- Protein: 9 g. (17%)
- Carbs: 3 g. (6%)

INGREDIENTS:

- 8 Jalapeno Peppers, split in half
- 150 grams Cream Cheese, softened
- 30 grams Shredded Cheddar Cheese
- 50 grams Cooked Bacon

PREPARATION:

Mix together cream cheese, grated cheddar, and bacon bits in a bowl.

Take each half of jalapeno and stuff with the cream cheese mixture.

Coat the fryer basket with non-stick spray.

Arrange stuffed jalapenos in the frying basket.

Cook for 5 minutes at 370F.

5. KETO ONION RINGS

Naturally sweet and juicy onion rings, wrapped in a crisp bacon crust. Skipping on the batter surely cut those carbs out of this recipe.

DETAILS:

- Preparation Time: 10 min
- Cooking Time: 8 min
- Serves: 4

NUTRITIONAL VALUES:

- Kcal per serve: 228
- Fat: 20 g. (78%)
- Protein: 7 g. (12%)
- Carbs: 6 g. (10%)

INGREDIENTS:

- 300 grams White Onion, sliced into rings
- 200 grams Bacon

PREPARATION:

Take each onion ring and wrap all round with a strip of bacon.

Arrange prepared onion rings in layers inside the frying basket using cooling racks.

Cook for 8 minutes at 380F.

6. PROSCIUTTO WRAPPED CHICKEN BITES

Juicy chicken thigh fillets, wrapped in prosciutto, then glazed in smoky maple syrup. These treats are just begging to be served at your next party.

DETAILS:

- Preparation Time: 10 min
- Cooking Time: 10 min

- Serves: 6

NUTRITIONAL VALUES:

- Kcal per serve: 224
- Fat: 8 g. (73%)
- Protein: 12 g. (21%)
- Carbs: 3 g. (6%)

INGREDIENTS:

- 300 grams Chicken Thigh Fillets, cut into bite-size pieces
- 150 grams Prosciutto
- Salt and Pepper to taste
- 1 tbsp Maple Syrup

PREPARATION:

Season chicken pieces lightly with salt an pepper.

Wrap each piece of chicken with a strip of prosciutto.

Arrange inside the frying basket and cook for 10 minutes at 370F.

Drizzle maple syrup before serving.

7. COCONUT AND CILANTRO CRUSTED SHRIMP POPPERS

Plump and tender shrimps in a flavorful crust of coconut shavings and fresh cilantro. This appetizer just sings tunes from the tropics in every bite.

DETAILS:

- Preparation Time: 5 minutes
- Cooking Time: 6 min
- Serves: 4

NUTRITIONAL VALUES:

- Kcal per serve: 246
- Fat: 20 g. (73%)
- Protein: 11 g. (19%)
- Carbs: 5 g. (8%)

INGREDIENTS:

- 300 grams Shrimp, peeled and deveined
- 100 grams Grated Coconut Meat
- 1 tbsp Chopped Cilantro
- 1 tbsp Lime Juice
- ¼ cup Butter
- ½ tsp Salt
- ½ tsp Turmeric Powder

- ¼ tsp Cayenne Pepper

PREPARATION:

Shake all ingredients in a bag making sure each piece of shrimp is evenly coated.

Arrange inside the frying basket and cook for 6 minutes at 400F.

8. MANCHEGO-STUFFED CHORIZO MEATBALLS

Smoky and full-flavored meatballs with a melty Manchego core. So much sophisticated flavor in something so simple to make.

DETAILS:

- Preparation Time: 15 minutes
- Cooking Time: 12 min
- Serves: 8

NUTRITIONAL VALUES:

- Kcal per serve: 175
- Fat: 14 g. (71%)
- Protein: 9 g. (21%)
- Carbs: 3 g. (8%)

INGREDIENTS:

- 300 grams Ground Pork
- 1 tsp Paprika
- 1 tsp Garlic Powder
- ¼ tsp Pepper
- ½ tsp Salt
- ½ tsp Dried Oregano
- 100 grams Manchego, diced
- 2 tbsp Butter, melted
- 100 grams Ground Almonds

PREPARATION:

Mix together pork mince, paprika, garlic powder, salt, pepper, and oregano. Divide into equal sized portions and roll into balls.

Stuff each ball with a cube of manchego in the center.

Brush meatballs with butter then roll in ground almonds.

Coat the fryer basket with non-stick spray.

Arrange meatballs inside and cook at

Cook for 12 minutes at 350F, turning halfway through the cooking time.

9. AIR FRYER PORK CHICHARRON

Pork belly cooked to a perfect brittle crisp. Definitely a keto-diet staple with absolutely no carbs!

DETAILS:

- Preparation Time: 5 minutes
- Cooking Time: 20 min
- Serves: 8

NUTRITIONAL VALUES:

- Kcal per serve: 324
- Fat: 33 g. (92%)
- Protein: 5 g. (8%)
- Carbs: 0 g. (0%)

INGREDIENTS:

- 500 grams Pork Belly, cut into 1" cubes

- Salt and Pepper, to taste

PREPARATION:

Season pork belly cubes with salt and pepper.

Transfer into the frying basket and cook at 400F for 20 minutes, flipping halfway through.

Season with a dash of salt and chili powder as desired.

10. TERIYAKI BACON AND ASPARAGUS BUNDLES

Roasted young asparagus spears bundled with strips of bacon, finished with a touch of teriyaki glaze for an interesting twist. Highly recommended!

DETAILS:

- Preparation Time: 10 minutes
- Cooking Time: 8 minutes
- Serves: 4

NUTRITIONAL VALUES:

- Kcal per serve: 235
- Fat: 20 g. (79%)

- Protein: 6 g. (11%)
- Carbs: 6 g. (10%)

INGREDIENTS:

- 300 grams Asparagus, trimmed
- 100 grams Bacon
- 2 tbsp Olive Oil
- Salt and Pepper, to taste

For the Teriyaki Glaze:

- 1 tbsp Soy Sauce
- 1 tbsp Mirin
- 2 tsp Honey
- 2 tsp Sesame Oil

PREPARATION:

Toss asparagus in olive oil, salt, and pepper.

Take 2-3 pieces of asparagus and bundle with a strip of bacon.

Arrange asparagus and bacon bundles inside the frying basket and cook for 8 minutes at 400F.

Whisk together all ingredients for the teriyaki glaze and drizzle over roasted asparagus.

MOUTH-WATERING SIDES

1. CHILI-PARMESAN ROASTED BRUSSELS SPROUTS

A truly savory way to prepare your brussels sprouts. These will come out so delicious you may want them for more than just a side.

DETAILS:

- Preparation Time: 10 minutes
- Cooking Time: 10 min
- Serves: 4

NUTRITIONAL VALUES:

- Kcal per serve: 264
- Fat: 23 g. (77%)
- Protein: 7 g. (10%)
- Carbs: 9 g. (13%)

INGREDIENTS:

- 250 grams Brussels Sprouts, cut into halves
- 50 grams Parmesan Cheese
- 50 grams Ground Walnuts
- ½ tsp Dried Chili Flakes
- ¼ cup Butter, melted
- pinch of Salt

PREPARATION:

Toss all ingredients in a baking pan.

Put pan in the air fryer and cook for 10 minutes at 350F, shaking to turn halfway through the time.

2. CAJUN-SPICED TURNIP STICKS

The neutral flavor of turnips served perfectly to showcase the bold Cajun flavors. A magnificent side to any grilled dish.

DETAILS:

- Preparation Time: 5 minutes
- Cooking Time: 10 min
- Serves: 3

NUTRITIONAL VALUES:

- Kcal per serve: 109
- Fat: 9 g. (76%)
- Protein: 3 g. (9%)
- Carbs: 4 g. (15%)

INGREDIENTS:

- 250 grams Turnips, peeled and cut into batons
- 2 tbsp Olive Oil
- 2 tsp Cajun Spice Mix
- pinch of Salt

PREPARATION:

Toss all ingredients in a baking pan.

Put pan in the air fryer and cook for 10 minutes at 350F, shaking to turn halfway through the time.

3. CURRIED OKRA CRISPS

Crisp air fried okra pieces with a spicy curry hazelnut coating. More to being a great side dish, this would be perfect for snacking or even as a vegan taco filling alternative.

DETAILS:

- Preparation Time: 5 min
- Cooking Time: 10 minutes
- Serves: 4

NUTRITIONAL VALUES:

- Kcal per serve: 160
- Fat: 14 g. (78%)
- Protein: 3 g. (6%)
- Carbs: 6 g. (16%)

INGREDIENTS:

- 200 grams Okra, chopped into 1.5" pieces
- 50 grams Hazelnuts, ground
- 2 tbsp Coconut Oil
- 1 tbsp Curry Powder
- ½ tsp Chili Powder
- ¼ tsp Salt

PREPARATION:

Toss all ingredients in a baking pan.

Put pan in the air fryer and cook for 10 minutes at 350F, shaking to turn halfway through the time.

4. RED MISO ROASTED EGGPLANTS

Red miso is infused in butter to give these roasted eggplants a deep umami richness. Perfect as a side, or even as a main dish if served with some warm poached eggs.

DETAILS:

- Preparation Time: 20 minutes
- Cooking Time: 10 min
- Serves: 4

NUTRITIONAL VALUES:

- Kcal per serve: 98
- Fat: 8 g. (74%)
- Protein: 2 g. (5%)
- Carbs: 5 g. (21%)

INGREDIENTS:

- 300 grams Japanese Eggplant, cut in half lengthwise
- 1 tbsp Red Miso Paste
- ¼ cup Butter, melted

PREPARATION:

Whisk together miso and butter.

Put eggplant halves in a resealable bag and pour in miso butter.

Seal and allow to marinate for 15 minutes.

Arrange eggplants in the frying basket and cook for 10 minutes at 350F.

5. ROASTED GREEN BEANS WITH ANCHOVIES AND CHEESE

Perfectly charred green beans with shallots, anchovies, and crumbled feta. Absolutely perfect with your favorite grilled dishes.

DETAILS:

- Preparation Time: 5 min
- Cooking Time: 10 min

- Serves: 3

NUTRITIONAL VALUES:

- Kcal per serve: 147
- Fat: 13 g. (77%)
- Protein: 5 g. (15%)
- Carbs: 3 g. (8%)

INGREDIENTS:

- 150 grams Green Beans
- 2 tbsp Olive Oil
- 30 grams Anchovies, chopped
- 1 tbsp minced Shallots
- pinch of Black Pepper
- ¼ cup Crumbled Feta

PREPARATION:

Toss all ingredients except for the feta cheese in a baking pan.

Put pan in the air fryer and cook for 10 minutes at 350F, shaking to turn halfway through the time.

Transfer to a serving platter and top with crumbled feta.

6. BACON-WRAPPED LEEKS

Chewy cookie dough balls with a nutty toasted coconut coating. It's good to know that these are low in carbs given how addictive they are.

DETAILS:

- Preparation Time: 10 min
- Cooking Time: 6 min
- Serves: 3

NUTRITIONAL VALUES:

- Kcal per serve: 124
- Fat: 10 g. (68%)
- Protein: 4 g. (11%)
- Carbs: 6 g. (21%)

INGREDIENTS:

- 100 grams Leeks, cut into 3" lengths
- 100 grams Bacon
- 1 tsp Balsamic Reduction

- pinch of freshly ground Black Pepper

PREPARATION:

Wrap leeks in strips of bacon. Season with freshly ground black pepper.

Arrange in the frying basket and roast for 10 minutes at 370F, rotating halfway through the time.

Transfer to a serving platter and drizzle balsamic reduction on top.

7. CHILI-GARLIC ASPARAGUS

Perfectly tender asparagus spears in a chili and garlic flavored butter. Good enough to make any simple dinner much more interesting.

DETAILS:

- Preparation Time: 5 minutes
- Cooking Time: 10 min
- Serves: 4

NUTRITIONAL VALUES:

- Kcal per serve: 117
- Fat: 12 g. (87%)

- Protein: 2 g. (4%)
- Carbs: 3 g. (9%)

INGREDIENTS:

- 250 grams Asparagus
- ¼ cup Butter, Melted
- 1 clove Garlic, minced
- ½ tsp Smoked Paprika
- ½ tsp Red Chili Flakes
- pinch of Salt

PREPARATION:

Toss all ingredients in a baking pan.

Put pan in the air fryer and cook for 10 minutes at 350F, shaking to turn halfway through the time.

8. AIR FRYER KALE CHIPS

Air-fried crisp kale chips with a smoky bbq taste. Yummy, easy, nutritious, keto, and vegan friendly. . . what more could you ask more?

DETAILS:

- Preparation Time: 5 minutes
- Cooking Time: 5 min
- Serves: 3

NUTRITIONAL VALUES:

- Kcal per serve: 117
- Fat: 9 g. (72%)
- Protein: 3 g. (7%)
- Carbs: 3 g. (21%)

INGREDIENTS:

- 200 grams Kale, stemmed
- 2 tbsp Olive Oil
- 1 tbsp Nutritional Yeast
- 1 tsp Garlic Powder
- ½ tsp Paprika
- ¼ tsp Salt,
- ¼ tsp Black Pepper

PREPARATION:

Toss all ingredients together in a bowl.

Arrange in the frying basket and cook for 5 minutes at 370F, shaking halfway through.

9. Air Fryer Zucchini Fries

A low-carb alternative to the typical side of fried potatoes. Perfect with just about anything for dinner.

DETAILS:

- Preparation Time: 5 minutes
- Cooking Time: 10 min
- Serves: 4

NUTRITIONAL VALUES:

- Kcal per serve: 158
- Fat: 7 g. (83%)
- Protein: 2 g. (6%)
- Carbs: 2 g. (11%)

INGREDIENTS:

- 250 grams Zucchini, cut into batons

- 2 tbsp Olive Oil
- 2 tsp Ranch Spice Mix
- pinch of Salt

PREPARATION:

Toss all ingredients in a bowl.

Put in the frying basket and cook for 10 minutes at 350F, shaking to turn halfway through the time.

10. BACON FAT ROASTED BUTTERNUT SQUASH

Tender and sweet roasted butternut squash with the smokiness of bacon and fragrance of sage. The taste and aroma of this humble side is simply remarkable.

DETAILS:

- Preparation Time: 5 minutes
- Cooking Time: 10 min
- Serves: 3

NUTRITIONAL VALUES:

- Kcal per serve: 107
- Fat: 8 g. (72%)
- Protein: 1 g. (2%)

- Carbs: 7 g. (26%)

INGREDIENTS:

- 200 grams Butternut Squash, cut into chunks
- 2 tbsp Bacon Fat
- 1 tsp Fresh Sage, chopped
- pinch of freshly ground Black Pepper

PREPARATION:

Toss all ingredients in a baking pan.

Put pan in the air fryer and cook for 10 minutes at 350F, shaking to turn halfway through the time.

QUICK AND EASY BREAKFAST RECIPES

1. AIR FRYER HAM AND LEEK FRITTATA

The smoky flavor of ham and natural sweetness of fresh leeks give unique life to this creamy frittata. With breakfast recipes such as this, you'll definitely look forward to the start of your day.

DETAILS:

- Preparation Time: 5 minutes
- Cooking Time: 20 min
- Serves: 4

NUTRITIONAL VALUES:

- Kcal per serve: 301
- Fat: 25 g. (74%)
- Protein: 15 g. (22%)
- Carbs: 3 g. (4%)

INGREDIENTS:

- 2 Whole Eggs
- 6 Egg Yolks
- ½ cup Heavy Cream
- 150 grams Smoked Ham, chopped
- ¼ cup Chopped Leeks
- pinch of Nutmeg
- ¼ tsp Salt

- ¼ tsp Black Pepper

PREPARATION:

Whisk eggs, heavy cream, and spices.

Spray a 7 inch round pan with non-stick cooking spray.

Add the chopped leeks and ham into the pan.

Pour egg mixture over the bacon and spinach.

Place the pan in the air fryer and cook for 20 minutes at 360F.

2. SMOKED SALMON AND SPINACH CASSEROLE

Celebrate with the flavors of the Caribbean in this truly festive pork belly specialty. Tender, juicy, and extremely flavorful!

DETAILS:

- Preparation Time: 5 hours
- Cooking Time: 20 min
- Serves: 3

NUTRITIONAL VALUES:

- Kcal per serve: 376
- Fat: 30 g. (70%)

- Protein: 22 g. (25%)
- Carbs: 5 g. (4%)

INGREDIENTS:

- 2 Whole Eggs
- 4 Egg Yolks
- ½ cup Heavy Cream
- ¼ cup Cream Cheese
- 150 grams Smoked Salmon, sliced
- 50 grams Frozen Spinach, chopped
- 1 tbsp Chopped Dill
- ¼ tsp Black Pepper

PREPARATION:

Whisk eggs, cream cheese, heavy cream, and black pepper.

Fold in the smoked salmon slices, spinach, and chopped dill.

Spray a 7 inch round pan with non-stick cooking spray.

Pour in the egg mixture.

Place the pan in the air fryer and cook for 20 minutes at 360F.

3. BACON AND TURKEY BREAKFAST CHILI

A turkey and bacon chili that's packed full of flavor. This will surely get you up and going for an active and busy day ahead.

DETAILS:

- Preparation Time: 5 min
- Cooking Time: 20 min
- Serves: 4

NUTRITIONAL VALUES:

- Kcal per serve: 300
- Fat: 24 g. (70%)
- Protein: 18 g. (23%)
- Carbs: 5 g. (7%)

INGREDIENTS:

- 200 grams Ground Turkey
- 200 grams Bacon, minced

- 1 cup Diced Tomatoes
- 1 cup Water
- ½ tsp Paprika
- ½ tsp Garlic Powder
- ½ tsp Cumin Powder
- Salt and Pepper, to taste

Toppings:

- ¼ cup Sour Cream
- ¼ cup Cheddar, grated
- 2 tbsp chopped Cilantro

PREPARATION:

Place the turkey mince and bacon in a pan. Place the pan inside the air fryer and cook for 5 minutes at 360F.

Stir in all remaining ingredients to the pan and cook for another 15 minutes, stirring halfway.

Ladle into bowls and top with sour cream, cheddar, and fresh cilantro.

4. AIR FRYER ZUCCHINI AND CHEESE QUICHE

A quick and light breakfast that's packed in nutrition. A smart and delicious way to fuel up your mornings.

DETAILS:

- Preparation Time: 10 min
- Cooking Time: 15 min
- Serves: 4

NUTRITIONAL VALUES:

- Kcal per serve: 263
- Fat: 21 g. (73%)
- Protein: 12 g. (20%)
- Carbs: 5 g. (7%)

INGREDIENTS:

- 3 Whole Eggs
- 3 Egg Yolks
- 100 grams Grated Zucchini
- ¼ cup Mexican Blend Cheese
- ½ cup Heavy Cream
- 1/3 cup Enchilada Sauce

- 1 tbsp Butter

PREPARATION:

Brush a 7 inch round pan with butter.

Whisk all remaining ingredients in a bowl and pour into the prepared pan.

Place the pan in the air fryer and cook for 20 minutes at 360F.

5. Air Fryer Vegetable Hash

Earthy brown mushrooms and crisp jicamas add substance to this creamy, cheesy breakfast hash. Healthy and indeed yummy.

DETAILS:

- Preparation Time: 5 min
- Cooking Time: 20 min
- Serves: 4

NUTRITIONAL VALUES:

- Kcal per serve: 362
- Fat: 31 g. (78%)

- Protein: 14 g. (17%)
- Carbs: 4 g. (5%)

INGREDIENTS:

- 5 Whole Eggs, beaten
- 1 cup Heavy Cream
- 50 grams Jicama, shredded
- 50 grams Brown Mushrooms, sliced
- 2 tbsp Diced Shallots
- ¼ cup Cheddar Cheese
- 2 tbsp Butter, melted
- 1 tsp Oregano
- ¼ tsp Salt
- pinch of Cayenne

PREPARATION:

Whisk the eggs and heavy cream in a bowl.

Fold in all remaining ingredients except for the butter.

Brush a round baking pan with melted butter. Pour in the egg mixture.

Place the pan in the air fryer and cook for 20 minutes at 360F.

6. Prosciutto and Blue Cheese Egg Cups

The briny and smoky flavor of prosciutto combined with the creamy pungency of blue cheese in a rich egg muffin. A delicious treat that's even more perfect on-the-go.

DETAILS:

- Preparation Time: 10 min
- Cooking Time: 12 min
- Serves: 4

NUTRITIONAL VALUES:

- Kcal per serve: 352
- Fat: 29 g. (75%)
- Protein: 17 g. (21%)
- Carbs: 3 g. (4%)

INGREDIENTS:

- 6 Whole Eggs

- 75 grams Prosciutto
- ¼ cup Crumbled Blue Cheese
- 1/2 cup Heavy Cream
- 1 tbsp Butter, melted

PREPARATION:

Whisk together eggs, heavy cream, and blue cheese in a bowl.

Brush silicon baking cups with melted butter.

Line each silicon cup with strips of prosciutto.

Pour egg mixture into the cups.

Put the filled cups into the fryer and cook for 12 minutes at 300F.

7. CHORIZO AND CREAM CHEESE PORTOBELLO CUPS

Juicy roasted portobello cups with a creamy minced chorizo filling. Definitely worth trying.

DETAILS:

- Preparation Time: 10 minutes
- Cooking Time: 8 min
- Serves: 4

NUTRITIONAL VALUES:

- Kcal per serve: 383
- Fat: 33 g. (77%)
- Protein: 16 g. (17%)
- Carbs: 6 g. (6%)

INGREDIENTS:

- 400 grams Portobello Mushrooms
- 200 grams Smoked Chorizo, minced
- 1/3 cup Cream Cheese
- 2 tbsp Chopped Spring Onions
- 2 tbsp Olive Oil
- Salt and Pepper, to taste

PREPARATION:

Mix cream cheese, minced chorizo, and chopped spring onions in a bowl.

Brush portobellos with olive oil. Slightly season with salt and pepper.

Fill each mushroom with cream cheese mixture.

Set mushrooms in the frying basket and cook for 8 minutes at 370F.

8. Air-Fried Keto Cheese Muffins

Finally, a low-carb option for all the muffin lovers out there! Unbelievably cheesy and flavorful for something that's totally guilt-free!

DETAILS:

- Preparation Time: 8 hours
- Cooking Time: 20 min
- Serves: 4

NUTRITIONAL VALUES:

- Kcal per serve: 232
- Fat: 19 g. (73%)
- Protein: 10 g. (17%)
- Carbs: 6 g. (10%)

INGREDIENTS:

- 300 grams Cauliflower, riced
- 50 grams White Onions, mixed
- 3 Egg Yolks

- 1 cup Cheddar Cheese, shredded
- ½ tsp Garlic Powder
- 2 tbsp Melted Butter
- ¼ tsp Salt

PREPARATION:

Mix all ingredients except for the butter in a bowl.

Brush silicone muffin molds with melted butter.

Fill molds with the cauliflower mixture.

Bake in the air fryer for 25 minutes at 350F.

9. JICAMA AND BACON HASH

A more flavorful alternative to your breakfast potato hash browns that's way lower in starch. Perfect for anytime-of-the-day snacking too.

DETAILS:

- Preparation Time: 10 minutes
- Cooking Time: 10 min
- Serves: 3

NUTRITIONAL VALUES:

- Kcal per serve: 448
- Fat: 38 g. (77%)
- Protein: 24 g. (22%)
- Carbs: 1 g. (1%)

INGREDIENTS:

- 150 grams Shredded Jicama
- 100 grams Bacon, chopped
- 2 tbsp Olive Oil
- 2 tbsp Chopped Parsley
- ¼ tsp Paprika
- ¼ tsp Salt
- pinch of Cayenne
- 2 Eggs

PREPARATION:

Mix together eggs, jicama, bacon, parsley, paprika, cayenne, and salt.

Form mixture into serving-sized patties.

Put olive oil in a pan and preheat in the air fryer at 400F.

Put in hash and cook for 4-5 minutes per side.

10. Air Fryer Sausage and Zucchini Latkes

Inspired by the popular Jewish staple, these breakfast hash by comparison packs a whole lot more flavor! Perfect on its own or as a patty for a healthier burger option.

DETAILS:

- Preparation Time: 10 minutes
- Cooking Time: 10 minutes
- Serves: 3

NUTRITIONAL VALUES:

- Kcal per serve: 266
- Fat: 22 g. (72%)
- Protein: 13 g. (19%)
- Carbs: 6 g. (9%)

INGREDIENTS:

- 150 grams Zucchini, spiralized
- 100 grams Sausage Mince
- 2 tbsp Olive Oil
- 2 tbsp Chopped Parsley
- ½ tsp Curry Powder
- ½ tsp Turmeric Powder
- ¼ tsp Salt
- 2 Eggs

PREPARATION:

Mix together eggs, zucchini, mince, parsley, curry powder, turmeric, and salt.

Form mixture into serving-sized patties.

Put olive oil in a pan and preheat in the air fryer at 400F.

Put in the latkes and cook for 4-5 minutes per side.

11. LOW-CARB AIR FRYER PANCAKES

Almond flour does the trick for this low-carb pancake recipe. Just as fluffy yet even more rich and yummy!

DETAILS:

- Preparation Time: 10 min
- Cooking Time: 15 min
- Serves: 4

NUTRITIONAL VALUES:

- Kcal per serve: 228
- Fat: 20 g. (79%)
- Protein: 9 g. (18%)
- Carbs: 2 g. (3%)

INGREDIENTS:

- ¼ cup Almond Flour
- 1 tsp Baking Powder
- ¼ tsp Salt
- 1 packet Stevia
- ¼ cup Heavy Cream

- ¼ cup Melted Butter
- 4 Eggs

PREPARATION:

Whisk together almond flour, baking powder, salt, and stevia in a bowl.

In a separate bowl, whisk together heavy cream, butter, and eggs.

Stir the dry mixture into the wet ingredients.

Coat a cast iron pan with non-stick spray. Set inside the air fryer and preheat for 5 minutes at 390F.

Pour in a serving of the pancake batter into the cast iron pan and cook for 6 minutes.

12. AIR FRYER BREAKFAST AVOCADOS

Bacon, egg, and melted cheese over a creamy roasted avocado half. Now we're talking breakfast.

DETAILS:

- Preparation Time: 5 min
- Cooking Time: 15 min

- Serves: 2

NUTRITIONAL VALUES:

- Kcal per serve: 425
- Fat: 36 g. (75%)
- Protein: 18 g. (17%)
- Carbs: 9 g. (8%)

INGREDIENTS:

- 1 Avocado, split in half and pitted
- 2 Eggs
- 4 strips Bacon
- ¼ cup Cheddar Cheese

PREPARATION:

Place avocados cut side up on a cutting board. Crack an egg into the cavity of each half.

Arrange strips of bacon on top.

Put prepared avocados into the frying basket and bake for 12 minutes at 400F.

Sprinkle shredded cheddar on top and bake for another 3 minutes.

13. SHAVED ASPARAGUS AND PARMA HAM HASH

Smoky parma ham and eggs in a nest of crisp asparagus shavings. Yummy, healthy, and low on carbs. . . perfect!

DETAILS:

- Preparation Time: 10 minutes
- Cooking Time: 10 min
- Serves: 3

NUTRITIONAL VALUES:

- Kcal per serve: 387
- Fat: 33 g. (75%)
- Protein: 16 g. (16%)
- Carbs: 8 g. (9%)

INGREDIENTS:

- 300 grams Asparagus, spiralized into flat ribbons
- 200 grams Parma ham, sliced
- 2 cloves Garlic, minced
- 3 Eggs
- 2 tbsp Olive Oil

PREPARATION:

Pour olive oil into a pan and preheat to 380F for 5 minutes in the air fryer.

Add the minced garlic, shaved asparagus, and parma ham slices in and cook for 5 minutes.

Stir and add the eggs in. Cook for another 3-5 minutes.

14. Bacon Wrapped Green Tomato Steaks

The popular recipe for fried green tomatoes gets a major upgrade with a layer of crisp bacon strips on the outside. Serve them up with a beautiful sunny-side-up and breakfast is done!

DETAILS:

- Preparation Time: 10 minutes

- Cooking Time: 25 min
- Serves: 3

NUTRITIONAL VALUES:

- Kcal per serve: 308
- Fat: 25 g. (69%)
- Protein: 15 g. (20%)
- Carbs: 9 g. (11%)

INGREDIENTS:

- 300 grams Green Tomatoes, sliced
- 150 grams Bacon
- 3 Fried Eggs for serving

PREPARATION:

Wrap tomato slices with strips of bacon.

Arrange in the frying basket and cook for 8 minutes at 400F, flipping halfway through.

Serve with fried eggs on top.

15. A IR F RYER C RAB O MELETTE

Sweet and delicate crabmeat in a creamy omelette. Surely a breakfast recipe to get all the seafood lovers excited.

DETAILS:

- Preparation Time: 10 minutes
- Cooking Time: 20 min
- Serves: 4

NUTRITIONAL VALUES:

- Kcal per serve: 251
- Fat: 21 g. (75%)
- Protein: 11 g. (19%)
- Carbs: 4 g. (6%)

INGREDIENTS:

- 2 Whole Eggs
- 6 Egg Yolks
- 4 tbsp Heavy Cream
- ¼ cup Canned Crab Meat
- 25 grams Corn Kernels
- 25 grams Frozen Peas

- 25 grams Red Bell Pepper, diced
- 2 tbsp Melted Butter
- ¼ tsp Salt
- ¼ tsp Black Pepper

PREPARATION:

Stir all ingredients in a bowl, except for the butter.

Brush a 7 inch round pan with melted butter.

Pour the egg mixture in.

Place the pan in the air fryer and cook for 20 minutes at 360F.

PORK AND BEEF MAIN MEALS

1. Air Fryer Crispy Pork Shank

Pork shanks made fall-off-the bone tender in an aromatic broth, then finished crisp in the air fryer. Serve with a side of slaw for a truly indulgent keto meal.

DETAILS:

- Preparation Time: 1 hour
- Cooking Time: 40 min
- Serves: 6

NUTRITIONAL VALUES:

- Kcal per serve: 326
- Fat: 20 g. (55%)
- Protein: 33 g. (44%)
- Carbs: 1 g. (1%)

INGREDIENTS:

- 1 Pork Shank, about 1 kilogram
- 6 Juniper Berries
- 6 cloves Garlic

- 1 Bay Leaf
- 6 Black Peppercorns
- 1 tsp Salt

PREPARATION:

Put all ingredients into a pressure cooker. Add enough water to get the contents fully submerged. Seal and cook on high pressure for 15 minutes. Allow pressure to release naturally.

Take pork shank out of the pot and leave to air dry for about and hour.

Rub more salt all around the pork shank.

Put pork shank in the frying basket and cook for 15 minutes at 400F.

2. Jerk-Marinated Pork Belly

Celebrate with the flavors of the Caribbean in this truly festive pork belly specialty. Tender, juicy, and extremely flavorful!

DETAILS:

- Preparation Time: 24 hours
- Cooking Time: 20 min

- Serves: 4

NUTRITIONAL VALUES:

- Kcal per serve: 444
- Fat: 44 g. (90%)
- Protein: 8 g. (8%)
- Carbs: 3 g. (2%)

INGREDIENTS:

- 500 grams Pork Belly, cut into 1" slices

For the Marinade:

- ¼ cup Lime Juice
- 50 grams Scallions, roughly chopped
- 4 Habanero Chilis, deseeded and chopped
- 4 cloves Garlic, crushed
- 2 Sprigs Fresh Thyme
- 30 grams Ginger, peeled and sliced
- 1 tbsp Brown Sugar
- 1 tsp Powdered All-Spice
- 1 tsp Black Pepper

PREPARATION:

Combine all the ingredients for the marinade in a blender. Process until smooth.

Put pork belly together with the marinade in a resealable bag. Squeeze out excess air and leave to marinate for 24-48 hours.

Take pork belly out of the bag, patting off any excess liquid. Leave in the chiller to dry out for at least 4 hours.

Put pork in the frying basket and cook for 10 minutes at 400F. Flip and continue roasting for another 7 minutes.

3. SALT AND PEPPER PORK RIBS

Chinese five-spice, gingers, and Szechuan chili give this pork rib dish an unforgettable Oriental flare. With less than a gram of net carbs per serving, this recipe may just be yummy to be considered healthy.

DETAILS:

- Preparation Time: 15 min
- Cooking Time: 15 min

- Serves: 4

NUTRITIONAL VALUES:

- Kcal per serve: 396
- Fat: 30 g. (68%)
- Protein: 29 g. (31%)
- Carbs: 1 g. (0%)

INGREDIENTS:

- 600 grams Pork Ribs, chopped into 2" pieces
- 2 tbsp Sesame Oil
- 1 tbsp Chinese Cooking Wine
- 1 tsp Chinese Five-Spice
- 1 tsp Minced Ginger
- 4 Szechuan Chilis, chopped
- 2 tbsp Melted Butter
- ½ tsp Salt

PREPARATION:

Toss pork ribs in sesame oil, cooking wine, five-spice, ginger, chilis, and salt. Marinate for at least 15 minutes.

Transfer ribs into the frying basket and cook for 10 minutes at 400F. Flip and continue roasting for another 7 minutes.

Toss ribs in melted butter and serve.

4. Keto Pork Saltimboca

Juicy pork tenderloin slices flavored with prosciutto and fresh sage. Literally translating to 'jumps in the mouth', this Italian saltimboca will surely please the palate.

DETAILS:

- Preparation Time: 10 min
- Cooking Time: 15 min
- Serves: 3

NUTRITIONAL VALUES:

- Kcal per serve: 456
- Fat: 35 g. (70%)
- Protein: 30 g. (28%)
- Carbs: 2 g. (2%)

INGREDIENTS:

- 300 grams Pork Tenderloin
- 200 grams Prosciutto
- 3 leaves Fresh Sage
- Salt and Pepper, to taste

For the Sauce

- ½ cup Chicken Stock
- 2 tbsp Butter
- 1 tsp Flour

PREPARATION:

Evenly slice pork tenderloin into three pieces. Take each slice and pound with a meat mallet until about half an inch thick. Season both sides with salt and pepper. Lay a leaf of fresh sage on top of the pork tenderloin and cover with strips of prosciutto. Pound lightly with a mallet to help the prosciutto adhere to the pork. Repeat for all slices of pork.

Arrange prepared pork in the frying basket. Cook for 10 minutes at 380F.

Heat butter in a pan then dust in the flour. Roast for about a minute. Whisk in chicken stock and drippings from the pork. Simmer until thick.

Pour sauce over the pork slices and serve.

5. PORK SHOULDER ROAST IN MADEIRA JUS

Perfectly succulent pork shoulder roast finished off with a smooth and refined Madeira gravy. Serve over some mashed cauliflower for a truly excellent low-carb dinner.

DETAILS:

- Preparation Time: 5 min
- Cooking Time: 25 min
- Serves: 4

NUTRITIONAL VALUES:

- Kcal per serve: 373
- Fat: 29 g. (71%)
- Protein: 23 g. (27%)
- Carbs: 2 g. (2%)

INGREDIENTS:

- 500 grams Pork Shoulder
- 1 cup Brown Stock
- ¼ cup Madeira Wine
- 2 tbsp Butter

- Salt and Pepper

PREPARATION:

Generously season pork with salt and pepper on all sides.

Put in the frying basket and cook for 20 minutes at 380F, flipping halfway through the cooking time.

Rest for 10 minutes before carving.

Meanwhile, whisk together roast drippings, brown stock, and Madeira in a pan. Simmer until reduced by half. Turn the heat off and whisk in cold butter nuggets.

Carve roast and serve with prepared jus.

6. Bacon and Parmesan Crusted Porkchops

Bacon bits and grated Parmesan replace breadcrumbs for crusting these crisp and juicy air fryer porkchops. Just as crisp, even more flavorful, and definitely low on the unwanted carbs.

DETAILS:

- Preparation Time: 10 min

- Cooking Time: 20 min
- Serves: 4

NUTRITIONAL VALUES:

- Kcal per serve: 399
- Fat: 31 g. (71%)
- Protein: 24 g. (26%)
- Carbs: 2 g. (2%)

INGREDIENTS:

- 400 grams Pork Chops
- ¼ cup grated Parmesan Cheese
- 70 grams Bacon Bits
- ½ tsp Paprika
- 1 tsp Garlic Powder
- ½ tsp Salt
- ¼ tsp Pepper
- 3 Egg Yolks

PREPARATION:

Mix together the bacon bits, parmesan, paprika, garlic powder, pepper, and salt in a bowl.

Dip the pork chops in egg yolks and coat evenly with the crust mixture.

Arrange pork in the frying basket and cook for 10 minutes per side at 380F.

7. AIR FRYER BBQ PORK RIBS

Moist, tender, sweet, spicy, and smoky. Just how bbq ribs are supposed to be!

DETAILS:
- Preparation Time: 8 hours
- Cooking Time: 20 min
- Serves: 4

NUTRITIONAL VALUES:
- Kcal per serve: 421
- Fat: 33 g. (71%)
- Protein: 25 g. (25%)
- Carbs: 5 g. (4%)

INGREDIENTS:
- 500 grams Pork Ribs, chopped into 2" pieces
- 2 tbsp Olive Oil

- 1 tbsp Soy Sauce
- 1 tsp Paprika
- 1 tsp Garlic Powder
- ½ tsp Salt
- ½ tsp Black Pepper
- 1 tbsp Liquid Smoke

For the Bbq Glaze

- ¼ cup Melted Butter
- 1 tbsp Low-Sodium Soy Sauce
- 1 tbsp Maple Syrup
- 1 tsp Cayenne

PREPARATION:

Toss pork ribs with olive oil, soy sauce, paprika, garlic powder, salt, pepper, and liquid smoke. Leave to marinate overnight.

Transfer ribs into the frying basket and cook for 10 minutes at 400F. Flip and continue roasting for another 7 minutes.

Whisk all the ingredients for the bbq glaze in a bowl. Toss in the cooked pork ribs until evenly coated.

8. Air Fryer Bulgogi Pork Chops

Succulent and tender pork chops that are extremely flavorful and unbelievably healthy. This bulgogi recipe alone proves why Korean cuisine is gaining so much popularity.

DETAILS:

- Preparation Time: 8 hours
- Cooking Time: 20 min
- Serves: 4

NUTRITIONAL VALUES:

- Kcal per serve: 388
- Fat: 30 g. (70%)
- Protein: 22 g. (24%)
- Carbs: 6 g. (6%)

INGREDIENTS:

- 400 grams Pork Chops(blade chops)

For the Marinade:

- 1 Pear, cored and roughly chopped
- 2 tbsp Gochujang

- 1 tbsp Brown Sugar
- ¼ cup Sesame Oil
- 2 tbsp Soy Sauce
- 30 grams Sesame Seeds
- 30 grams Spring Onions
- 20 grams Ginger

PREPARATION:

Combine all ingredients for the marinade in a blender. Process until smooth.

Put the porkchops in a resealable bag and pour in the marinade. Squeeze out excess air and leave to marinate in the chiller overnight.

Take pork chops out of the marinade and arrange in the frying basket.

Cook at 380F for 20 minutes, flipping halfway through the cooking time.

9. Air Fryer Rib Eye Steak with Blue Cheese Butter

Pungent and rich blue cheese butter served over a perfectly done rib eye steak. Yummy. . . enough said.

DETAILS:

- Preparation Time: 10 minutes
- Cooking Time: 8 min
- Serves: 3

NUTRITIONAL VALUES:

- Kcal per serve: 448
- Fat: 38 g. (77%)
- Protein: 24 g. (22%)
- Carbs: 1 g. (1%)

INGREDIENTS:

- 400 grams Rib Eye Steak
- Salt and Pepper, to taste

For the Compound Butter:

- ¼ cup Butter, room temperature
- 2 tbsp Blue Cheese
- ¼ tsp Ground Black Pepper
- 1 tsp Lemon Juice

PREPARATION:

Whisk butter until light and airy. Stir in the blue cheese, pepper, and lemon juice. Wrap in cling film and leave in the freezer to solidify.

Pat steaks dry and season with salt an freshly ground black pepper.

Cook steaks for 4 minutes per side at 400F.

Slice compound butter and top on hot rib eye steaks.

10. LOW-CARB AIR FRYER BEEF JERKY

Beef jerkies could have been the perfect low-carb snack if not for the high sugar content in most commercial choices. This recipe solves that problem so we can all enjoy snacking free of guilt.

DETAILS:

- Preparation Time: 8 hours
- Cooking Time: 1 hour
- Serves: 6

NUTRITIONAL VALUES:

- Kcal per serve: 243
- Fat: 14 g. (54%)

- Protein: 18 g. (32%)
- Carbs: 8 g. (14%)

INGREDIENTS:

- 500 grams Beef Round, thinly sliced

For the Marinade:

- ½ cup Soy Sauce
- ¼ cup Worcestershire Sauce
- ½ cup Swerve Granular Sweetener
- 1 tsp Cayenne
- 1 tsp Onion Powder
- 1 tsp Garlic Powder
- 1 tsp Smoked Paprika
- 1 tbsp Liquid Smoke

PREPARATION:

Whisk together all ingredients for the marinade.

Put the slices of beef together with the marinade in a resealable bag. Marinate in the chiller overnight.

Arrange the beef slices in the air fryer in layers using cooling racks.

Cook for an hour at 180F.

11. Bacon-Wrapped Filet Mignon

Melt-in-your-mouth tender filet mignon steaks flavored and kept extra moist by strips of smoky bacon. This has become the king of steaks for obvious reason.

DETAILS:

- Preparation Time: 10 min
- Cooking Time: 8 min
- Serves: 2

NUTRITIONAL VALUES:

- Kcal per serve: 524
- Fat: 41 g. (70%)
- Protein: 35 g. (28%)
- Carbs: 3 g. (2%)

INGREDIENTS:

- 300 grams Beef Tenderloin
- 100 grams Bacon
- Salt and Pepper, to taste

PREPARATION:

Season filet mignon steaks with salt and pepper on both sides.

Wrap each steak with bacon strips, securing with toothpicks as needed.

Arrange steaks in the frying basket and cook for 4 minutes per side at 400F.

12. Keto Swedish Meatballs

An equal mix of beef and pork mince ensure to keep these meatballs from cooking out tough to the bite. With only a gram of carbs per serving, these meatballs are well worth adding to your keto-recipe library.

DETAILS:

- Preparation Time: 10 min
- Cooking Time: 10 min
- Serves: 6

NUTRITIONAL VALUES:

- Kcal per serve: 291
- Fat: 24 g. (76%)
- Protein: 15 g. (22%)

- Carbs: 1 g. (2%)

INGREDIENTS:

- 250 grams Ground Beef
- 250 grams Ground Pork
- ¼ cup Almond Flour
- ½ cup Cream
- 1 Egg
- 1 tsp Onion Powder
- ½ tsp Ground All-Spice
- ½ tsp Pepper

PREPARATION:

Mix all ingredients in a bowl. Form into equal-sized balls.

Coat the frying basket with non-stick spray.

Arrange the meatballs inside and cook for 10 minutes at 370F, flipping the meatballs halfway through.

13. AIR FRYER TRI-TIP ROAST WITH CILANTRO CHIMICHURRI

Deeply-flavored tri-tip roast out of the air fryer. Those tender slices of beef get even better with a pairing of the bright cilantro chimichurri.

DETAILS:

- Preparation Time: 8 hours
- Cooking Time: 45 min
- Serves: 6

NUTRITIONAL VALUES:

- Kcal per serve: 307
- Fat: 24 g. (71%)
- Protein: 18 g. (25%)
- Carbs: 4 g. (4%)

INGREDIENTS:

- 500 grams Tri-Tip Roast
- 4 cloves Garlic, crushed
- 1 tbsp Cumin Powder
- ¼ cup Lime Juice
- 1 tsp Salt

- 1 tsp Ground Black Pepper
- ¼ cup Olive Oil

For the Chimichurri

- ¼ cup Olive Oil
- ¼ cup Red Wine Vinegar
- 1 tbsp minced Shallots
- 1 clove Garlic
- ½ cup chopped Cilantro
- Salt and Pepper, to taste

PREPARATION:

Combine the roast, garlic, cumin, lime juice, olive oil, pepper, and salt in a resealable bag. Leave in the chiller overnight to marinate.

Blend all ingredients for the chimichurri in a food processor. Set aside.

Take tri-tip out of the bag, shaking off any excess marinade.

Put in the frying basket and cook for 45 minutes at 360F.

Rest for 10 minutes.

Carve and serve with chimichurri on the side.

14. AIR FRYER MEATLOAF

Who doesn't love a juicy slice of homemade meatloaf? Easy, filling, yummy, and with only a gram of carbs in this recipe... keto-friendly.

DETAILS:

- Preparation Time: 10 minutes
- Cooking Time: 25 min
- Serves: 6

NUTRITIONAL VALUES:

- Kcal per serve: 290
- Fat: 25 g. (78%)
- Protein: 14 g. (21%)
- Carbs: 1 g. (1%)

INGREDIENTS:

- 500 grams Ground Beef
- ¼ cup Almond Meal
- 2 tbsp Butter
- 3 Egg Yolks
- 1 tbsp chopped Fresh Thyme

- 1 tsp Onion Powder
- ½ tsp Pepper

PREPARATION:

Combine all ingredients in a bowl. Mix until thoroughly combined.

Transfer mixture into a baking pan.

Set pan in the frying basket and cook for 25 minutes at 390F.

Let the meatloaf rest for 10 minutes before slicing.

15. CRISP BEEF RIBS WITH SESAME VINAIGRETTE

Tender and juicy beef ribs, marinated in Oriental spices. Even goes with a dipping sesame vinaigrette for more Asian flavor.

DETAILS:

- Preparation Time: 8 hours
- Cooking Time: 35 min
- Serves: 3

NUTRITIONAL VALUES:

- Kcal per serve: 440

- Fat: 33 g. (68%)
- Protein: 28 g. (27%)
- Carbs: 6 g. (5%)

INGREDIENTS:

- 400 grams Beef Ribs
- 2 tbsp Soy Sauce
- 2 tbsp Rice Wine Vinegar
- 1 tsp Minced Ginger
- ¼ cup Chopped Spring Onions
- 2 stalks Lemongrass, chopped

For the Sesame Vinaigrette:

- 2 tbsp Soy Sauce
- 1 tbsp Lime Juice
- 2 tbsp Sesame Oil
- 1 tsp Grated Ginger
- 2 tsp Honey

PREPARATION:

Combine the beef ribs, soy sauce, rice wine vinegar, ginger, spring onions, and lemongrass in a resealable bag. Marinate overnight.

Transfer the beef ribs to the frying basket and cook at 400F for 10 minutes. Reduce temperature to 320F and cook for another 25 minutes.

Whisk all ingredients for the vinaigrette.

Slice beef ribs into segments and serve with vinaigrette on the side.

TASTY POULTRY RECIPES

1. Crisp Chicken Thigh Adobo

Chicken thighs made extremely savory by coconut vinegar and garlic marinade, then finished succulent and crisp in the air fryer. This dish alone has brought Filipino cuisine to the world food map.

DETAILS:

- Preparation Time: 4 hours
- Cooking Time: 20 min
- Serves: 3

NUTRITIONAL VALUES:

- Kcal per serve: 386
- Fat: 31 g. (73%)
- Protein: 22 g. (25%)
- Carbs: 2 g. (2%)

INGREDIENTS:

- 400 grams Chicken Leg Quarters
- 3 cloves Garlic, crushed
- ¼ cup Coconut Vinegar

- 1 tbsp Soy Sauce
- 2 Dried Bay Leaves
- 6 Black Peppercorns
- 1 tsp Salt
- 2 tbsp Coconut Oil

PREPARATION:

Marinate chicken legs in coconut vinegar, crushed garlic, soy sauce, bay leaves, black peppercorns, and salt for at least 4 hours.

Take chicken out of the marinade and leave to come to room temperature.

Toss chicken in coconut oil.

Arrange in the frying basket and cook for 10 minutes at 350F.

Flip and cook for another 10 minutes.

2. AIR-FRYER CHICKEN CORDON BLEU

Mouth-watering layers of juicy chicken thigh, smoky ham, and Gruyere cheese in every bite! This version of a popular French dish uses almond flour in place of bread crumbs to cut down on the carbs.

DETAILS:

- Preparation Time: 15 min
- Cooking Time: 16 min
- Serves: 4

NUTRITIONAL VALUES:

- Kcal per serve: 402
- Fat: 31 g. (70%)
- Protein: 26 g. (28%)
- Carbs: 2 g. (2%)

INGREDIENTS:

- 300 grams Chicken Thigh Fillets
- 150 grams Sliced Ham
- 100 grams Gruyere Cheese, shaved
- ¼ cup Melted Butter
- 1/2 cup Almond Flour
- ½ tsp Italian Seasoning
- Salt and Pepper, to taste

PREPARATION:

Butterfly chicken thighs and flatten with a meat mallet.

Take a piece of prepared chicken thigh. Season with salt and pepper on both sides then stuff with sliced ham and gruyere cheese. Fold over and secure with toothpicks.

Whisk together almond flour and Italian seasoning.

Brush both sides of the stuffed chicken thighs with melted butter and dredge in the seasoned flour mixture.

Repeat for remaining ingredients.

Arrange prepared chicken thighs in the frying basket and cook at 350F for 8 minutes per side.

3. AIR-FRYER ROASTED PERI-PERI CHICKEN

A Portuguese favorite done right in your very own kitchen. Smoky, tangy, spicy. . . highly recommended!

DETAILS:

- Preparation Time: 5 min
- Cooking Time: 13 min

- Serves: 6

NUTRITIONAL VALUES:

- Kcal per serve: 505
- Fat: 41 g. (73%)
- Protein: 28 g. (24%)
- Carbs: 4 g. (3%)

INGREDIENTS:

- 1 Kilogram Chicken, chopped
- 4 cloves Garlic, crushed
- 4 Red Chilis, deseeded and chopped
- 1 Lemon, juice and zest
- 1 Orange, juice
- 1/2 cup Olive Oil
- 1 tbsp Paprika
- 1 tsp Salt
- ½ tsp Black Pepper

PREPARATION:

Combine all ingredients except for the chicken in a blender. Process until smooth.

Put chicken pieces in a resealable bag. Pour in the marinade and gently massage to coat chicken pieces evenly. Seal and leave to marinate in the chiller overnight.

Take chicken pieces out of the marinade and arrange in the frying basket.

Cook at 350F for 10 minutes per side.

4. Chili-Hoisin Chicken Wings

An Asian twist on everyone's chicken wing favorite. The Oriental flavor of hoisin pair up with the subtle heat of Sri Racha for a truly unique buffalo wing experience.

DETAILS:

- Preparation Time: 5 min
- Cooking Time: 30 min
- Serves: 3

NUTRITIONAL VALUES:

- Kcal per serve: 477
- Fat: 37 g. (71%)
- Protein: 30 g. (27%)
- Carbs: 2 g. (2%)

INGREDIENTS:

- 400 grams Chicken Wings, split at the joint
- Salt and Pepper, to taste

For the Glaze

- 2 tbsp Sri Racha
- 1 tbsp Hoisin Sauce
- ¼ cup melted Butter

PREPARATION:

Lightly season chicken pieces with salt and pepper.

Arrange in the frying basket and cook for 24 minutes at 380F, flipping halfway.

Increase temperature to 400F and bake for another 5 minutes.

Whisk all ingredients for the glaze in a bowl.

Toss chicken wings in the glaze until evenly coated.

5. Hazelnut Crusted Turkey Fingers

Tender strips of turkey breast in a nutty crust of hazelnuts and thyme. A perfect light snack that's high in protein but low in carbs.

DETAILS:

- Preparation Time: 5 min
- Cooking Time: 13 min
- Serves: 3

NUTRITIONAL VALUES:

- Kcal per serve: 468
- Fat: 36 g. (67%)
- Protein: 33 g. (30%)
- Carbs: 4 g. (4%)

INGREDIENTS:

- 400 grams Turkey Breast Fillets, cut into strips
- 3 tbsp Melted Butter
- 75 grams Ground Hazelnuts

- ½ tsp Dried Thyme
- ½ tsp Salt
- ¼ tsp Pepper

PREPARATION:

Mix together ground hazelnuts, dried thyme, salt, and pepper in a bowl.

Pat turkey strips dry with paper towels then toss in the melted butter.

Coat evenly with the ground hazelnut mixture.

Arrange in the frying basket and cook at 350F for 8 minutes per side.

6. Bacon-Wrapped Turkey Breast with Dijon Butter

Air fryer turkey breasts made perfectly moist and rich by smoky strips of bacon. The dijon compound butter in the end just makes the dish even more juicy and flavorful.

DETAILS:

- Preparation Time: 10 min
- Cooking Time: 40 min

- Serves: 6

NUTRITIONAL VALUES:

- Kcal per serve: 353
- Fat: 29 g. (70%)
- Protein: 23 g. (26%)
- Carbs: 3 g. (4%)

INGREDIENTS:

- 500 grams Turkey Breast
- 200 grams Bacon
- 1 stick Butter
- 1 tbsp Dijon Mustard
- 2 tsp Worcestershire Sauce
- 1 tbsp Chopped Sage
- Salt and Pepper, to taste

PREPARATION:

In a bowl, whisk butter until pale-colored and slightly airy. Fold in dijon mustard, worcestershire sauce, chopped sage, salt, and pepper. Wrap mixture in cling film and freeze to solidify.

Wrap turkey breast with strips of bacon.

Put in the frying basket and cook for 20 minutes at 350F. Flip and cook for another 20 minutes.

Carve turkey breast and top with slices of prepared dijon butter.

7. Air Fryer Chicken Tandoori

Perfectly juicy and smoky chicken legs done without all the hassles from setting up a live charcoal grill. And that garlic-tahini dipping sauce. . . delicious!

DETAILS:

- Preparation Time: 4 hours
- Cooking Time: 20 min
- Serves: 4

NUTRITIONAL VALUES:

- Kcal per serve: 418
- Fat: 41 g. (70%)
- Protein: 33 g. (26%)
- Carbs: 6 g. (4%)

INGREDIENTS:

- 500 grams Chicken Leg Quarters, split at the joints

- 1 cup Full-Fat Yogurt
- 2 tbsp Tandoori Paste
- Salt and Pepper, to taste

For Dipping

- ½ cup Mayonnaise
- 2 tbsp Tahini
- 2 tsp Lemon Juice
- 1 clove Garlic, grated
- Salt and Pepper, to taste

PREPARATION:

Whisk together all ingredients for the dipping sauce. Set aside.

Whisk together yogurt and tandoori paste in a bowl. Toss in chicken pieces and leave to marinate in the chiller for at least 4 hours.

Take chicken out of the marinade and arrange in the frying basket.

Cook for 10 minutes per side at 350F.

Serve with the garlic-tahini dipping sauce.

8. Garlic Parmesan Chicken Nuggets

Ground walnuts make up for a low-carb substitute to bread crumbs in this keto-friendly chicken nugget recipe. Just as crisp but even more tasty and healthy.

DETAILS:

- Preparation Time: 5 min
- Cooking Time: 15 min
- Serves: 4

NUTRITIONAL VALUES:

- Kcal per serve: 356
- Fat: 28 g. (70%)
- Protein: 21 g. (26%)
- Carbs: 3 g. (4%)

INGREDIENTS:

- 400 grams Chicken Thigh Fillets, cut into chunks
- ½ cup Walnuts, ground
- ¼ cup Grated Parmesan
- 3 Egg Yolks
- 2 cloves Garlic

- 1 tbsp Chopped Parsley
- Salt and Pepper, to taste

PREPARATION:

Mix together ground walnuts, parmesan, parsley, salt, and pepper.

Beat egg yolks with about 2 tablespoons of water.

Season chicken pieces with salt and pepper, dip in egg yolks, and roll in the crumb mixture.

Arrange nuggets in the frying basket and cook for 7 minutes per side at 350F.

9. Asian-Style Air Fryer Rotiserrie Chicken

A simple rotisserie chicken in the air fryer with a twist of Asian flavors. The annatto oil gives a unique earthy profile that balances out the pungency of ginger and garlic while giving the roast a beautiful golden sheen.

DETAILS:

- Preparation Time: 8 hours
- Cooking Time: 40 min
- Serves: 6

NUTRITIONAL VALUES:

- Kcal per serve: 662
- Fat: 62 g. (83%)
- Protein: 24 g. (16%)
- Carbs: 1 g. (1%)

INGREDIENTS:

- 1 whole Spring Chicken(approx. 800 grams)
- ¼ cup Lime Juice
- 2 cups Diet Lime Soda
- 30 grams Ginger, thinly sliced
- 4 cloves Garlic, crushed
- 8 Black Peppercorns
- 2 stalks Lemongrass, thinly sliced
- ¼ cup Annatto Oil
- Salt, to taste

PREPARATION:

Combine chicken, lime soda, lime juice, ginger, garlic, black peppercorns, and lemongrass in a resealable bag. Leave overnight in the chiller to marinate.

Take chicken out of the bag and pat dry with paper towels. Brush with annatto oil and season generously with salt.

Set chicken breast side up in the frying basket.

Cook at 350F for 25 minutes.

Flip chicken and baste with more annatto oil. Cook for another 25 minutes.

www.ingramcontent.com/pod-product-compliance
Lightning Source LLC
Chambersburg PA
CBHW071440070526
44578CB00001B/161